MY BRAIN **STILL** NEEDS
GLASSES

Project Editor: Marianne Prairie
Art Direction & Design: Christine Hébert
Graphic Design: Chantal Landry
Translation: Matthew Brown
Editing & revision: Alison Ramsey
Proofreading: Robert Ronald
Illustrations: Nadia Berghella

EXCLUSIVE DISTRIBUTOR:

For Canada and the United States:
Simon & Schuster Canada
166 King Street East, Suite 300
Toronto, ON M5A 1J3
phone: (647) 427-8882
          1-800-387-0446
Fax: (647) 430-9446
simonandschuster.ca

Bibliothèque et Archives nationales du Québec
and Library and Archives Canada cataloguing in
publication

Title: My brain still needs glasses : ADHD in adults /
Annick Vincent.
Other titles: Mon cerveau a encore besoin de
lunettes. English
Names: Vincent, Annick, 1965- author.

Description: 4th edition. | Translation of:
Mon cerveau a encore besoin de lunettes.
Identifiers: Canadiana (print) 20220012946 |
Canadiana (ebook) 20220012954 |
ISBN 9781988002965 | ISBN 9781988002972
(EPUB)
Subjects: LCSH: Attention-deficit disorder in adults.
| LCSH: Attention-deficit disorder in adults—
Treatment. | LCSH: Attention-deficit disorder in
adults—Genetic aspects.
Classification: LCC RC394.A85 V5613 2022 |
DDC 616.85/89—dc23

01-23

© 2014, 2016, Les Éditions Québec-Livre

© 2017, 2023, Juniper Publishing,
division of the Sogides Group Inc.,
a subsidiary of Québecor Média Inc.
(Montreal, Quebec)

Legal deposit: 2023
National Library of Québec
National Library of Canada

ISBN 978-1-988002-96-5

Conseil des Arts   Canada Council
du Canada   for the Arts

We gratefully acknowledge the support of the Canada
Council for the Arts for its publishing program.

Financé par le gouvernement du Canada | **Canadä**
Funded by the Government of Canada

We acknowledge the financial support of the
Government of Canada through the Canada Book
Fund for our publishing activities.

Annick Vincent, MD

MY BRAIN **STILL** NEEDS
GLASSES

ADHD IN ADOLESCENTS AND ADULTS

A Practical and Friendly Guide for People Living
with Attention Deficit Hyperactivity Disorder

**4th
edition**

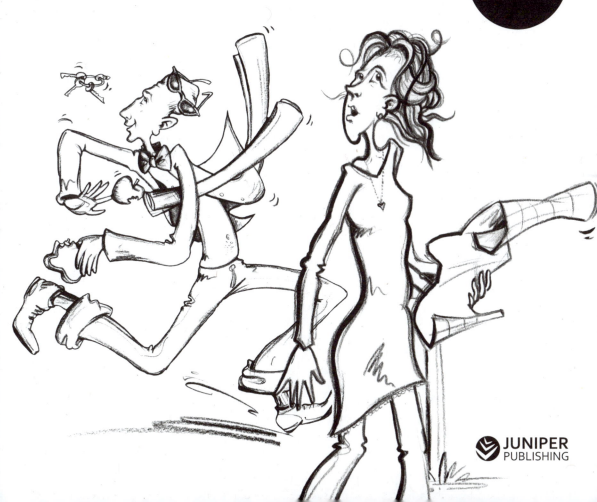

JUNIPER PUBLISHING

Preface

Dr. Vincent has revised, expanded, updated and enhanced her landmark book *My Brain STILL Needs Glasses*. It is a "must-read" text for anyone whose life has been touched by ADHD! Clearly and engagingly written, it provides a comprehensive, broad-ranging consideration of all aspects of ADHD from childhood through adolescence and adulthood. It incorporates testimonies of patients coping with the disorder, scientific findings and clinical approaches, and practical tools to improve daily life and make ADHD less of an impairing disorder.

I've long admired Dr. Vincent for her creative insights into the many dimensions of ADHD. Her genuine enthusiasm for the subject, her deep regard for her patients, and her clinical wisdom fills each page of the book. It contains important new information from neuroscience, neuropsychology, and clinical psychiatry presented in a highly readable and straightforward fashion. It is insightful, compassionate, humorous and practical. It offers hope as well as insights and solutions for those whose lives have been challenged by having ADHD.

BRAVO and THANK YOU, Dr. Vincent!

Anthony Rostain
Psychiatrist

Preface

My Brain STILL Needs Glasses is an accessible book that presents the most up-to-date research on ADHD among adults in a clear and simple style. It focuses on diagnostic and therapeutic approaches and the role of medication among the proven strategies to successfully deal with ADHD, for those affected as well as for those around them.

Annick Vincent has a unique set of skills. She is a sensitive and experienced clinician who understands ADHD in adulthood, both from a doctor's and patient's perspective. She's an expert in the medical literature in the field. Lastly and most importantly, she combines all of this with the ability to explain complex ideas in simple but clear language.

There have always been children, adolescents and adults with ADHD. However, it's only recently that we've come to understand how this condition affects people and what strategies can help. Today, people with ADHD can better understand their own experience and the options available to them. It's my view that doctors can rely on this book to provide their patients and their families with sound and balanced information.

Margaret Weiss
Psychiatrist

TABLE OF CONTENTS

A word from the author

A big thank-you to the adults with Attention Deficit Hyperactivity Disorder (ADHD) who shared their stories, struggles and triumphs with me. It is thanks to you that the project for the children's book *My Brain Needs Glasses* was born; and it is for you and with your help that this second book, aimed at adolescents and adults, was conceived and created.

A warm thank-you to the practitioners in the field, the friends and families, the health care professionals and the scientists who, each in their own way, try to better understand the complexity of this neurodevelopmental disorder and find solutions that work.

The scientific approaches described in this book are the subject of consensus among a Canadian group of experts of which I am a part (CADDRA). I invite the reader to consult the most recent edition of the *Canadian ADHD Practice Guidelines*, available on the website caddra.ca. I would like to thank the experienced and devoted professionals for their work and dedication in helping persons with ADHD and those who support them on their journey.

A thousand thank-yous to everyone who believed in this project and who continue to offer their support and advice. A very special thank-you to my husband, children, family, friends and colleagues. Your support, your ideas and your enthusiasm have been and always will be very precious to me.

This book is titled *My Brain STILL Needs Glasses* for many reasons.

ADHD is a neurological disorder that manifests itself during childhood with symptoms of inattention and/or hyperactivity/impulsivity, and for some, emotional hyperreactivity. The various methods used to reduce the symptoms and their impacts act like a "pair of glasses for the brain" by helping to improve concentration. They allow better self-control, whether it be for focus, fidgetiness, behavior or emotions. I chose the image of "psychological glasses" to describe the non-pharmaceutical strategies, and "biological glasses" to describe the effects of ADHD medication.

My first book, *My Brain Needs Glasses*, explains to children, in a playful manner, with accompanying illustrations, what ADHD is and what types of "glasses for the brain" are available. Because more than half of all children with ADHD will continue to have symptoms once they become adolescents and adults, the book you're now holding is aimed at grown-ups looking for tools, reliable and scientifically grounded information and stories of other people's experiences with ADHD.

The three testimonials that open this book were told to me by adults whom I've had the privilege of knowing and helping. Each of them found their "pair of glasses" and have chosen to share their experience with ADHD. The other testimonials are inspired by real experiences. The names and certain details, however, have been modified to preserve the anonymity of the sources.

This book is addressed to everyone: to the parents who are watching their child grow up with ADHD; to the adolescents and adults who are wondering about the condition; to the adult who has been living with ADHD since childhood; to the many people who want to better understand the reality of ADHD so that they can help someone they know.

I invite you to take an adventure, with this book as your guide, on a journey filled with fascinating pathways and discoveries that are as important as they are exciting.

Good reading and bon voyage!

Annick Vincent
Psychiatrist

Personal stories from adults living with ADHD

For as long as I can remember, distraction, procrastination, lack of self-confidence and difficulty sleeping were problems I had to deal with on a daily basis. In my twenties, my family doctor discovered I have ADHD, and urged me several times to get treatment. For a long time I resisted, for various reasons, including misconceptions I held about the role of medication. I thought that option was only for people in desperate situations. I was a mother of two, a university graduate who worked in management positions and made a good salary. Nothing seemed to justify taking medication that I then thought was just a crutch. I saw taking pills as something to be ashamed of, a sign of weakness. I was even proud of doing without them — all I had to do was force myself to pay attention better!

I compensated by fighting against myself on a daily basis, trying not to forget appointments or lose my keys and credit cards, to resist erupting in anger and the constant need for stimulation, to stop making unrealistic schedules and being hopelessly disorganized. In other words, I was battling all the hallmarks of ADHD. I tried to maintain a sense of humor to keep my colleagues and loved ones laughing, to take the drama out of my many slip-ups. Throughout these years, I never thought I needed to learn more about ADHD. I didn't know I was suffering from a neurobiological disorder that can't be regulated merely by making an effort — no matter how massive that effort is.

I was convinced that the symptoms would diminish as I got older, but in fact, the opposite was true. When I turned 50, I faced a new professional challenge: joining a great company with a good team and a hyperstimulating environment. I underestimated what an effect working in an open space for the first time would have. My brain was constantly bombarded and distracted. I compensated by working extra hours in the evenings and on weekends to make sure I always got good results. On top of that, I was dealing with a lot of personal stress. Exhausted, I spent my free time trying to get organized, and I doubted myself constantly. I felt like I was having memory loss, and I was always questioning my own actions. Rather than seeing my symptoms diminish as I'd hoped, I realized I had hit a wall. That's how I ended up — worn out, extremely anxious and very emotional — in my doctor's office.

My doctor immediately recognized that my untreated ADHD had contributed to my deteriorated state. A colleague happened to send me a text about ADHD around the same time, and I saw myself in it quite clearly. I couldn't deny it any longer. I was suffering so badly! I couldn't see any solution but to try the medication my doctor recommended. I agreed to start on the adventure under the supervision of a medical specialist in the field. The medication led to a significant and fast reduction in the intensity of the symptoms of ADHD. However, above all it was the global approach proposed by Dr. Annick Vincent (a healthy lifestyle, tools and medication) that made me realize that for years my behavior had been specifically related to ADHD, and could have been attenuated to a great degree if I hadn't always been in a state of denial. I finally understood that drugs are neither magic nor evil, and that I could improve my life by adapting and changing my habits.

Today I'm at peace with myself. Things in my life are less intense and I haven't become any less effective. In fact, for the first time in my life I feel I can access my true potential. I'm full of energy. I feel less like I'm caught in a whirlwind; my loved ones and my colleagues don't have to suffer the consequences of my problem as much. I have better self-esteem. I can now try to live in the present moment, because my mind isn't always trying to take me somewhere else.

Now that I know the benefits of proper treatment, I will always regret not having confronted ADHD earlier. I want to help fight the taboos and prejudices that still surround ADHD, and encourage everyone who suffers from the condition to get help from health care professionals so they can learn more about the negative effects, but also about the treatments and tools available to control the disorder, and open up the space for the positive side of their personality!

Marie, age 53

Since my early childhood, I have been living with the consequences of ADHD. When I was young, in addition to being inattentive, I was hyperactive. My parents have told me that they got to know the neighborhood by running after me! I was diagnosed with ADHD when I was about four years old. My parents, who didn't really understand the side effects, didn't think it was a good idea to use medication to reduce my symptoms. My school years were absolute hell: bad behavior, constant agitation, forgetting many details in my schoolwork, etc.

Since I had a pretty volatile personality, the consequences on my social life were substantial. I had low self-esteem, mostly because I couldn't form bonds with my peers. My adolescence was punctuated by heartbreak and family, social, and personal disappointments. When I was about 20, everything spiralled downwards: I was diagnosed with major depression and experienced significant episodes of anxiety. After many medical consultations, I was referred to a psychiatric center that specialized in ADHD. Clearly, my ADHD symptoms had begun to weigh heavily upon me. Once the diagnosis was made, I was given a prescription first for one medication, then for another. Unfortunately, they didn't particularly help me. Recently, a trial with a different medication has given me much relief.

This tool, or "pair of biological glasses," allows me to adequately control my impulsiveness, my lack of attention and my "hyperactive" memory. Now, I want to start psychotherapy to help me get to another level and to improve day-to-day life with ADHD.

Mathieu, age 25

· · · · · · · · · · · · · · ·

When I think about it, I was always a "last minute" kind of guy. On the other hand, this never seemed to be a big problem for me. When I settled down to work, the internal pressure pushed my system into high gear. The adrenaline allowed me to work 24 hours without a break and to finish the job on time.

But after undergoing an operation that required a long convalescence, everything seemed to have changed. My return to work rapidly turned into a nightmare. As soon as I tried to work, I was invaded by a thousand thoughts that had nothing to do with the task at hand... At first, I tried to reason with myself, to make an effort to concentrate on what I had to do, but I just couldn't do it.

So, I felt this pressure slowly developing deep inside me. Then it became physically perceptible. I felt palpitations. I became a ball of energy. I felt like I was full of intense energy that was spinning in a void. No amount of reasoning could break through the mental paralysis that these phenomena produced. The results were always the same: I left my desk without having done anything productive. I felt more and more useless and incompetent... In short,

I was having dark thoughts about my future on this planet more and more often.

My wife suggested that I get help. After several fruitless attempts, I met with a psychologist who aroused my suspicions about ADHD. She was the one who put me on the right track, which finally allowed me to get the professional help I needed.

Clearly, my problems haven't disappeared by magic. Now, if I want to have a life worth living — a productive life — I have to think about how to manage my energy. Luckily, I have a new "pair of biological glasses" that helps balance me better, and I can count on a good support system.

André, age 58

Myths and realities

Even though they may have the best intentions in the world, some people still have preconceived notions about Attention Deficit Hyperactivity Disorder. Let's explore a few points.

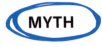 **ADHD is a new disease invented by the medical establishment.**

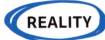 There are descriptions of cases of agitated and inattentive children in scientific literature going back more than a century. In the early 20th century, scientists were already proposing the hypothesis that these abnormal behaviors weren't controlled at will, but were linked to neurological problems. It was during the 1930s that doctors noticed that amphetamines reduced the intensity of ADHD symptoms.

Until the late '80s, doctors paid more attention to the motor symptoms (fidgetiness and impulsivity) than to the cognitive aspects of ADHD — the less visible but extremely important impacts of this condition. In the last decades of the century, genetic research and longitudinal follow-up studies were done with cohorts of young people with ADHD as they grew into adulthood. This research continues today. It was also at that time that researchers started looking at the cognitive difficulties associated with ADHD such as distractibility, forgetfulness, procrastination, difficulty getting started and scattered attention.

Since the start of the '90s, new technology has helped us acquire new knowledge about how the brain develops and functions. It has demonstrated that **the brain of a person with ADHD develops and functions differently**. Nonetheless, these technologies are not used as diagnostic tools.

MYTH **ADHD is a consequence of parental neglect, and the term describes the behavioral problems of badly raised children.**

REALITY We don't know the exact causes of ADHD. However, scientific studies have shown that ADHD is a neurodevelopmental problem that is transmitted from one generation to the next. It has nothing to do with how children are raised. In the majority of cases, it is genetically transmitted, somewhat like height, eye and hair color. Rarely do neurological events which have occurred — during pregnancy or delivery, for example, or due to infections or brain trauma — result in the same clinical picture. While genetics is certainly involved in the causal factors of ADHD, the current state of knowledge on the subject does not make it possible to use genetic testing to support a diagnosis of ADHD or to predict which treatment will be most effective.

The way children with ADHD are raised and educated will greatly influence who they become as adults. Support, or the absence of support, influences the development of self-esteem and can mitigate the risks of anxiety, depression and substance abuse. Family and friends also have an impact on the intensity of behavioral problems associated with ADHD. An encouraging, understanding and stimulating environment promotes personal development and helps to reduce the impacts and obstacles associated with the daily burden of ADHD. If a person with ADHD has good intellectual and emotional resources, he or she will also have an advantage in developing, implementing and maintaining effective adaptive techniques to reduce the intensity of the difficulties associated with the condition.

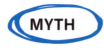 **MYTH** **ADHD only affects children and disappears before they reach adulthood.**

REALITY During the '80s, the scientific community proposed the hypothesis that the symptoms of ADHD were secondary to delayed brain development. According to this notion, ADHD symptoms should disappear as the neurons matured before reaching adulthood. This perception was contradicted by follow-up studies published during the '90s, in which children with ADHD were re-evaluated as adults. They showed that for many, fidgetiness and agitation did, in fact, become less intense and easier to channel with age. However, impulsivity and attention problems frequently remained a problem beyond the age of 20.

Some statistics

Epidemiological studies have shown that **ADHD is present in about 5% of children.** The levels vary between 2% and 12%, depending on the criteria used and the region studied. Most follow-up studies have demonstrated that **the symptoms of ADHD persist in more than half of the adults** who were diagnosed as children. Clinicians and researchers now agree that the impact of ADHD remains significant in the daily life of many adults. The results of a U.S. study from 2006 estimated that **4% of the general population of adults is affected with ADHD**. At the time of this epidemiological study, less than 10% of these adults were diagnosed or treated, and at least half had consulted a doctor for a mental health problem. The ratio of boys to girls is between **9:1** and **3:2.** In adults, the ratio is approximately **3:2.** Boys with ADHD are often more agitated and exhibit more behavioral problems than do girls with ADHD, who are often more inattentive. That may explain why affected boys are detected earlier and more easily than are affected girls.

We now know that access to a diagnosis and adequate treatment is as important for adults as it is for young children. ADHD research for every stage of life is flourishing today. However, many people today still suffer from a lack information, inadequate training of educators and health care workers and a lack of resources for the diagnostic assessment and treatment of ADHD.

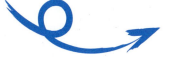

GOOD TO KNOW

Canadian psychiatrists and pioneers in the field

Drs. Lily Hechtman, Gabrielle Weiss and Margaret Weiss were pioneers in the study of children with ADHD who have grown into adulthood. Their publications have added a major contribution to the work of other researchers around the world and have advanced our understanding of the different faces of ADHD at each stage of life. Their work has helped experts provide diagnostic criteria that can create a better picture of ADHD in adults (DSM-5[1]).

1. *Diagnostic and Statistical Manual of Mental Disorders*, Fifth Edition (DSM-5), American Psychiatric Association, Washington DC, 2013.

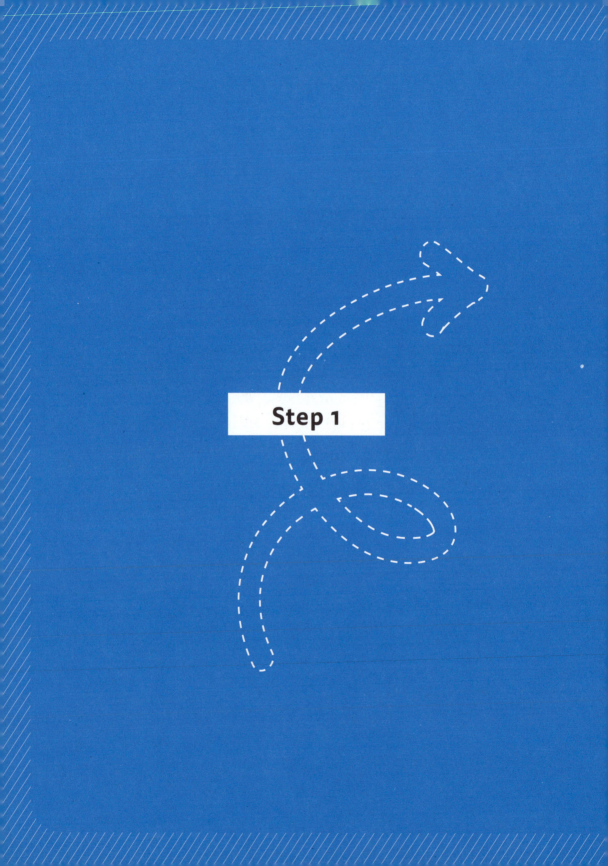

Step 1

UNDERSTANDING
ADHD

> **Symptoms and
> clinical presentations**

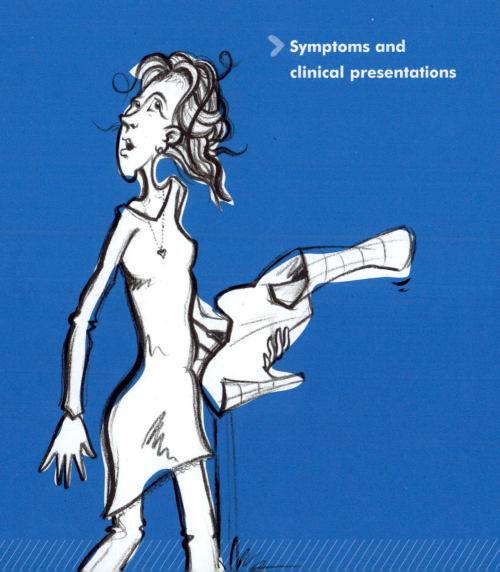

Many people in different circumstances experience symptoms of inattention, agitation or impulsivity. Not everyone who gets spaced out or moves around a lot has ADHD! To see things clearly, let's start by defining the different types of attention and exploring the factors that modulate our attentional capacity. Then we'll proceed to look at the different manifestations of ADHD and their expression over the course of a lifetime.

A brief exploration of attention

Paying attention could be defined as the action of centering our mental activity on a specific thing. In our daily lives, we use the term "concentration" to designate the act of voluntarily paying attention to something. This requires a varying amount of mental effort depending on the type of task, our motivation level and the conditions we're under in the moment we execute that attentional task. In contrast, what is known as "floating attention" is a cognitive process that's more spontaneous, and is carried out in an automatic mode. It demands less mental effort and is less sensitive to disruptive factors. Let's distinguish some forms of attention as they are characterized within neuropsychology.

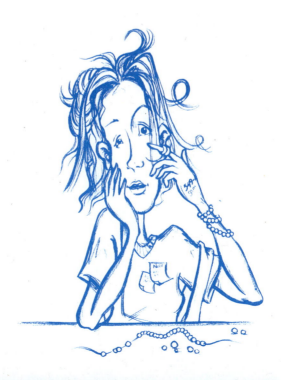

Sustained attention

Sustained attention allows us to concentrate on the same task for long periods of time, even if it is monotonous and prolonged.

> **Examples:** An air traffic controller who watches a blank screen, waiting to see an object appear or move. A factory worker who examines products that pass by on a conveyor belt, looking for manufacturing defects.

Divided (or shared) attention

Divided or shared attention allows us to execute multiple tasks at the same time. Effective "multitasking" is possible only by cutting each task into mini-steps and performing each separately. Divided attention helps us move from one task to another while maintaining a minimal level of attention on all fronts.

> **Examples:** A parent who, while preparing a meal, keeps an eye on the children, while also talking on the phone. A salesperson who is talking to their client and is thinking about the profit on the sale, all the while calculating the "best price" on his calculator.

Selective attention

Selective attention allows us to focus on one particular task while ignoring other stimuli that could distract us.

> **Examples:** A person following a conversation in a crowded room. A child listening to their teacher, even though they can see other students playing on the playground outside the window and has fleeting thoughts about last summer's vacation. A worker staying focused on a presentation despite seeing an email notification.

Recognizing the factors that influence our attention span

Various factors affect our ability to modulate our attention. They can sometimes make it seem like we are dealing with ADHD ("Pseudo-ADHD") or complicate that condition if we do have it. Some of these factors are environmental, some are related to the task itself and some are components of our individual capacities for attention.

Noises, visual stimuli, bodily perceptions and ideas all compete to draw our attention. Our interest in a task and our motivation are major driving forces that stimulate and maintain our attention. Someone who's tired or feeling overwhelmed by emotion will not be able to focus effectively on the task at hand. The same goes for someone who's disorganized, neglects their health practices or takes medication or consumes toxic substances that impair the brain's functioning. If you find you have problems with attention, it is important to identify the causes, and also to target the elements that can improve your brain's functioning and the elements that can reduce its effectiveness — regardless of whether you suffer from ADHD!

FACTORS that can MIMIC ADHD (PSEUDO-ADHD) or AGGRAVATE IT

Energy: Fatigue, cognitive overload, health problems

Emotions: Stress, emotional overload (anxiety/sadness/anger)

Organization: Lack of routine and structure, poor time and space management

Lifestyle: Poor diet, sleep problems, lack of physical activity, poorly controlled use of screen time

Toxicity: Side effects from medication, consumption of toxic substances

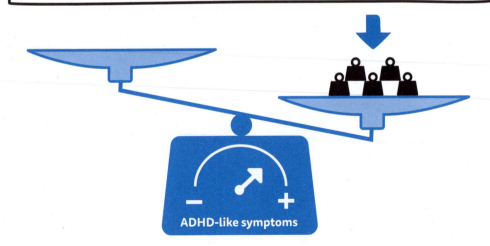

ADHD-like symptoms

Taking care of your brain is part of taking care of yourself!

ADOPT HEALTHY HABITS

Our brain needs to be in shape! When our lifestyle choices are poor, it's no surprise that we develop symptoms that resemble ADHD, or that symptoms worsen for those of us who live with it. ADHD or not, it is essential to have good sleep and nutrition habits, to be active and organized to better resist distractions in our environment — including screens (Internet, social and video games). Be careful: brain at work! Avoid taking medications that have sedative effects, or saturating neurons with alcohol or drugs.

MAXIMIZE YOUR ENERGY

Our brain needs rest. It is important to address issues that hamper recovery or drain energy, whether it is lack of sleep, a health condition or task overload. We often charge forward, obsessed with "doing" while forgetting to "be." We need to recharge our batteries by introducing moments of mindful presence into our day, learning to include planned breaks, allowing ourselves periods of relaxation amid the whirlwind, and moderating our pace to preserve our energy. These are challenges that should not be ignored!

OPTIMIZE YOUR ORGANIZATION

Our brain needs support. When we let routines slide, or lose control of our time and structure to our day, the resulting disorganization hinders our ability to effectively self-manage. We can arrange our environment in ways that reduce distracting stimuli and keep us feeling comfortable as we work. Prioritize tasks according to cognitive load as well as available energy and time. And, finally, arm ourselves with reminders to supplement our memory and jot down good ideas rather than letting them slip away!

TAME YOUR EMOTIONS

Our brain needs calm and tranquility. When our train of thought is hijacked by strong emotions like anxiety, sadness or anger, our brain devotes much of its resources to try to manage the emotional overload: it can no longer work efficiently. Young or old, we benefit from recognizing the waves of emotions that overwhelm us, so that we can discover how to ground ourselves and adjust our reaction by stepping back and identifying what is causing the disturbance. Our ideas and emotions are ephemeral. Let's learn to observe them without judgment, remembering that, like clouds that hide the sun, they will eventually pass.

FUEL YOUR MOTIVATION

Our brain needs encouragement. It's easy to get lost when the beacon that lights our way flickers or dies. Are we guided by what makes sense to us, by our deepest values? Are those who accompany us kind? And are we kind to ourselves? Let's pay attention to our sources of motivation. Let's channel our strengths and pinpoint our unique challenges. Let's identify our obstacles, accept being helped and share our burden. Progress is made when we welcome change and when we dare to explore, lose our balance, stumble and get up again. Progress is also made when we recognize mistakes as a learning opportunity and learn to choose our path as well as those who share it.

A word from the author

Repetitive or chronic stress and its associated anxiety are a major source of attentional difficulties and can contribute to many mental and physical health problems.

Resilience is our ability to bounce back from stress. According to the work of Rachel Thibeault, a Canadian occupational therapist, and her collaborators, resilience is developed like a muscle, through the daily repetition of intentional actions that nourish us and carry meaning. On an individual level, the activities of Centering, Contemplation, Creativity or Creation, Contribution, and Connectedness are our allies, both in our everyday lives and during more turbulent times. On a collective level, Rachel Thibeault uses the acronym HERMES to highlight elements of a caring environment that promote resilience. H: Do I feel heard? E: Do I feel equipped? R: Do I feel recognized? M: Do I feel my work has meaning? E: Do I feel treated equitably? S: Do I feel safe and supported?

I have developed my own acronym to help me take care of myself. I want to share it with you:

CARPE DIEM
Contact (with the self, with others and with the world)
Attention (focused and kind)
Resilience
Participation
Enchantment

Dynamism
Inspiration
Expectation
Movement

It's up to you to discover your own guiding principles. Enjoy the journey!

Unmasking ADHD

ADHD is a neurological problem that is often genetically transmitted and first manifests itself in childhood through **difficulties modulating** thoughts (inattention), movements and behavior (hyperactivity/impulsivity). Difficulty modulating emotions (hyperreactivity) could often be added to this list. The symptoms are not the result of a lack of will, but a lack of ability. Therapeutic strategies aim to increase a person's capacity to self-modulate and reduce the impacts of ADHD so the individual can reach their full potential.

To help people understand the symptoms of ADHD, let's compare the flow of information in the brain to road network traffic. Studies on the functioning of the brain in people with ADHD have revealed difficulties at the level of what psychologists call executive functions. These functions are responsible for self-modulation: the capacity to initiate, inhibit or amplify thoughts, movements, behaviors and emotions. You could think of executive functions like traffic police, controlling stopping, braking, changes of direction and "right of way" for stimuli, ideas, movements, actions and even, in some cases, emotions. In the brain of people with ADHD, it has been proven that this network for transmitting and modulating information needs a higher level of stimulation to prioritize signals effectively and to keep things going in the right direction. It's as if the traffic lights and road signs are missing and the cars don't have good accelerators or brakes.

For a person who "lacks brakes," the thought with top priority is usually the most recent one to arrive. It pushes the preceding thoughts out of the way, no matter how pertinent they may have been. That's what some people call **restless** or **"bumper-car"**

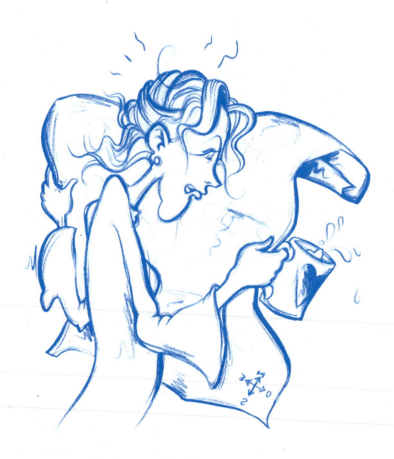

thoughts. Sounds, images or situations can provoke a new idea and initiate a new project that replaces the last one the person was engaged in. The person's efforts are scattered, and they have a hard time finishing what they started. They move too fast, don't pay enough attention and end up losing track of things, making careless mistakes along the way and forgetting what they are doing. So, many of these people will talk about how they misplace things, no matter how important they may be, because they are unable to focus on the present moment. Finding information in the memory's labyrinth is harder for a person with ADHD, especially if there are no clues (like memos) or visual reminders for reference. Anything not in the field of vision tends to disappear from their mind...and disappear from the physical world! This explains why many keep things in plain sight when they don't want to forget them; the result is cluttered table-tops, counters and even floors!

The main symptoms of ADHD

Now let's explore the different portraits of ADHD (its different symptoms) and see how they can affect daily life (i.e., examine their functional impacts), as well as how age can influence the expression of ADHD. In later sections we will discuss the diagnostic approach, adaptive strategies to better cope with ADHD and specific treatments for the condition.

People with ADHD are born with the condition and grow up with it. Some who present ADHD in childhood continue to manifest the symptoms after the age of 18. In all cases, the symptoms appear early in life; the impacts, however, can appear later. The symptoms of ADHD can become more visible and debilitating in adolescence or adulthood, when the compensatory mechanisms stop allowing the individuals to cope.

About 70% of people living with ADHD deal every day with the impacts associated with the triad of **inattention, hyperactivity and impulsivity**; while others suffer mainly from attentional difficul-

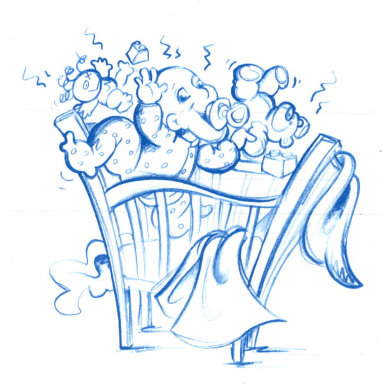

ties, with no significant symptoms of hyperactivity/impulsivity. The latter condition is commonly known as ADD. For people with this condition, hyperactivity is concentrated in the realm of ideas. Often "spaced out," lost in thought and struggling to take action, to get started and finish tasks on time, these people don't fit in with the traditional picture of hyperactivity associated with ADHD. Attentional symptoms are less visible, mainly because they are less intrusive for others than fidgeting and impulsivity; so diagnosis often takes place later in life.

The inattention/hyperactivity/impulsivity triad

The **distractibility** component consists of a high sensitivity to distracting stimuli, restless thoughts and difficulty establishing priorities, organizing and planning, and starting and finishing tasks. Inattentive people get scattered easily and lose track of their ideas. During conversations or presentations, they have difficulty taking notes, make lots of errors due to distraction ("careless mistakes") and have to read, reread and double-check. Many of them have learned to counter forgetfulness with organizational tools like memos, lists and agendas with reminders. Unlike children, adults with ADHD don't lose things: they temporarily misplace them or take a ridiculous amount of time finding them. Many speak of a tendency to wait until the last minute to perform tasks that don't inspire them or that require sustained attentional effort. Often, they become more effective at the last minute, when they are stimulated by a sense of pressure and urgency. This can have consequences on their personal, academic or professional life. The energy and extra time required to compensate for distraction and to get reorganized can also lead to exhaustion and even a loss of alertness, which can result in falling asleep while reading, for instance.

> *It's as if I have a telephone operator in my head. She manages dozens of telephone lines at the same time, cutting the connection and passing from one conversation to another without my permission.*
>
> Anne, age 45

> *It's as if someone else has a remote control for my thoughts and is zapping from one channel to another: even if I'm interested in an idea, it is pushed away by the next one.*
>
> Benoit, age 32

In the realm of ADHD, **hyperactivity** can manifest as abrupt, sudden or poorly controlled movements. People often describe a feeling like having a vibrating motor inside them that's always running or that's hard to turn off. They have difficulty staying still when they're supposed to, they can't put on the brakes, they move and speak too quickly. Because the same mechanisms are activated to stop mental restlessness AND physical restlessness, it is important to realize that people affected by ADHD **need to move to think effectively!** Simply stopping to go to sleep at night is a feat. People affected often describe feeling "jet lag" in the morning. It's hard for them to wake up, they feel foggy-headed and their start-up system is slow. As they grow up, individuals with hyperactivity learn to deal with physical restlessness and channel it into their work and, for some, sports. Many athletes with ADHD will tell you that physical activity helps them function better in their daily lives. Manifestations of restlessness become subtler with age and emerge when affected people are in a situation where they have to wait or stay still. They no longer bounce off the walls but can remain seated; however, they say they still have a higher need to keep moving, as if driven by a motor. Staying still — "putting on the brakes" — takes a lot of energy. Waiting is uncomfortable, and moving helps them stay alert. They tap, doodle, hum, chew gum, overtly or subtly move their hands and feet, balance on their chair or fidget with whatever's in their hands.

Impulsivity can manifest as irritability while waiting in line or driving and as a tendency to interrupt. Adults with ADHD tend to be better able to contain their impatience and express it less explosively than when they were children. However, regardless of age, impulsivity in a person's words, decisions and actions can have impacts on all spheres of life.

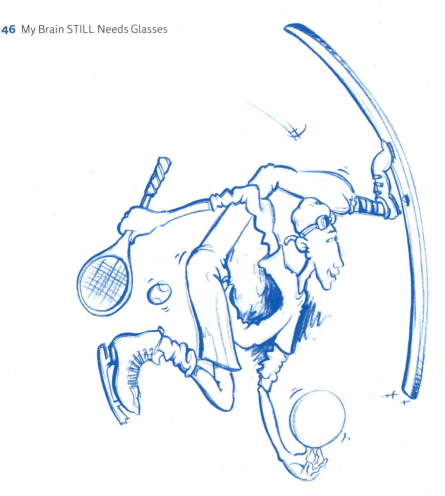

Emotional hyperreactivity

In young and old alike, the difficulty with self-control that is intrinsic to ADHD can have repercussions on emotion management. This problem is less well-known, but it's extremely important to understand. Emotional reactions may be appropriate to the context, but are felt and expressed more intensely and with fewer filters. People describe feeling edgy, hypersensitive or irritable. Emotions come in powerful waves that are hard to contain. Joyous peaks and crashes of anger or tears happen intermittently. In quick response to an event, ideas and emotions start to collide, and the individual is helpless to control them. They don't have the ability to step back and begin an inner dialogue, and are less able to modulate their reactions. **They don't act; they react, or rather, hyper-react.** They want to put on the brakes and contain themselves so they don't erupt, but it's extremely hard. The process is exhausting in the long run. This phenomenon is often disorienting for those around them; it appears as a kind of excess and can cause interpersonal conflicts. When it comes to finding therapeutic strategies, it's important to recognize that this mood rollercoaster may be related to ADHD and not to a personality nor a mood disorder such as Bipolar Disorder.

Ever since I was a little girl, I've been called "Spacey Sophie". I never caused problems in class. My teachers found me calm — even too calm. They often called on me to bring me back to Earth. I missed explanations and, embarrassed, I ended up not daring to ask questions because I had heard the response "I just said that, Sophie. Where were you?" so many times. I worked hard, but in spite of my efforts, I almost failed English class and I had a lot of problems in math. I have a miserable time getting organized and I'm scatterbrained. Simply choosing what clothes to wear in the morning is a challenge. The disorder in my room and in my things is legendary. My parents wonder how I'm going to handle things when I'm on my own.

Recently, my cousin Matthew was diagnosed with combined ADHD — both inattention and hyperactivity. My mother thinks that I'm a lot like him, without the fidgetiness. I read about ADHD and learned that, in fact, there are people who have ADHD with only symptoms of inattention. When I saw that Matthew was doing better with his medications, I decided to consult my doctor. He told me that he wanted to do a full neuropsychologic work-up because of my difficulties at school. It took a while, but I finally finished all the tests. I was surprised to learn that I had an above-average IQ! The doctor also confirmed that I had the predominantly inattentive type of ADHD. I will meet with him next week and we will discuss possible treatments. I hope that I will do better.

Sophie, age 16

When ADHD gets complex

Being spaced out, disorganized, overly agitated or impulsive can be a detriment to different aspects of life. In most cases, ADHD is associated with other problems that can make diagnosis complicated and daily life harder. These problems must be taken into account when it comes to finding treatment strategies. For some individuals, these symptoms are the most visible ones, those that push them to seek help. Detecting the underlying ADHD can be a complex matter when its presentation is tainted by other problems.

Educational difficulties and learning disorders

It is possible to have ADHD without having difficulties at school. Usually, people with ADHD who don't have academic problems end up seeking professional help because of functional impacts on other aspects of their life. For many, however, ADHD may impair learning capacities. When this is the case, the risk of interrupting or dropping out of school is greater.

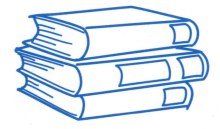

Here is a list of difficulties in school that may be related to ADHD:
- ▷ difficulty paying attention and making a sustained mental effort
- ▷ answering questions impulsively, without having finished reading the statement or question
- ▷ making errors due to distraction when writing and answering questions
- ▷ writing too quickly and messily, and having problems with spelling or grammar: forgetting letters, reversing letters or making punctuation errors
- ▷ having difficulty reading properly and following the thread, finding, extracting or synthesizing information
- ▷ taking incomplete class notes due to difficulty paying attention to what the teacher is saying
- ▷ having difficulties in mathematics, skipping steps in problem solving or having problems doing mental calculations
- ▷ managing study periods ineffectively due to difficulty planning and getting organized and procrastination
- ▷ running out of time during exams because reading, reflecting, answering questions and rereading takes more time
- ▷ falling behind because of difficulty undertaking a particular task; lack of organization or forgetfulness
- ▷ losing or misplacing materials or homework; backpack and work area are so chaotic that it's difficult to find anything
- ▷ getting inconsistent results and being seen as distracted, lazy or lacking motivation

Different elements can influence the learning process and academic results. It's important to distinguish learning problems associated with ADHD from specific Learning Disorders (LD). Learning Disorders may come in the form of difficulties understanding written or oral language, or specific problems with reading, writing or mathematics (dyslexia, dysorthographia, dyscalculia). Identifying these problems makes it possible to implement adequate strategies to help students get on the path to success (see *Support at school*, page 144).

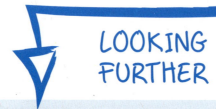

LOOKING FURTHER

Specific Learning Disorders: essential specialists

Even though navigating the consultation process can be complex, it's a worthwhile task: diagnostic assessment and clarification can guide the individual and equip them with different intervention strategies adapted to their situation. Here are a few elements that may help.

For significant academic difficulties — particularly if a Learning Disorder, an intellectual deficiency or giftedness are suspected — it is recommended to have the clinical investigation completed by a school psychologist or a neuropsychologist, regardless of whether the individual has received a diagnosis of ADHD or Autism Spectrum Disorder (ASD). Neuropsychological tests make it possible to assess higher cognitive functions like intellectual quotient, attentional abilities, executive functions and memory.

An assessment conducted by a speech therapist can detect the presence of an oral language and/or speech disorder. These include dysphasia (a primary language impairment), dyspraxia (a motor development impairment affecting writing and more), as well as dyslexia and dysorthographia (specific language impairment). Specific interventions may be proposed depending on the type of language disorder identified.

If the individual presents motor difficulties that interfere with learning (for example, in writing), a consultation with an occupational therapist is recommended.

Services offered by special education teachers and specialized teachers will give the individual tools to use in their education. Look for resources that are available in your area.

Difficulty maintaining a healthy lifestyle

ADHD often results in **sleep problems**. A great many affected adults report that since childhood they have had difficulty sleeping at night; it's hard to "turn off their brain." For some, mental or physical restlessness prevents sleep, while others don't feel sleepy, or resist the feeling. Many procrastinate to avoid going to sleep, preferring more stimulating activities like watching movies, surfing the Internet or using social media. The result is fewer hours of sleep, which only worsens the symptoms of ADHD the next day!

When they do get to sleep, some affected individuals say they sleep soundly, but others manifest hyperactivity during the night. Sleep is often described as non-restorative, and many people may have a hard time getting out of bed in the morning. Sleep apnea is more common among people with ADHD and should be detected as soon as possible, since the health consequences can be severe.

The biology regulating the circadian rhythm of sleep and wakefulness is different in many individuals with ADHD. This helps explain why they fall asleep later: studies have shown that they experience a later release of melatonin, one of the messengers that prepares the brain for sleep. Exposure to light is another factor that delays this phenomenon. It is therefore essential for individuals having difficulties sleeping to reduce brightness in the evening and shut off all screens at least an hour before going to bed.

Recent studies show that a lack of sleep and ADHD itself increase the risk of **obesity**. Other factors contribute to that risk, such as difficulty planning and preparing meals (leading to the consumption of fast food and junk food) and the tendency to skip meals and eat impulsively. Sedentariness is certainly another factor, but this is amplified by excessive time spent in front of screens (social media, Internet surfing and gaming) and difficulty organizing one's day in order to find time for physical activitiy.

Oppositional behaviors and Conduct Disorders

ADHD in young people is often associated with a behavioral disorder called Oppositional Defiant Disorder (ODD). ODD usually tends to diminish with age. It's common that adults still describe difficulties with relationships to authority figures and tend to be obstinate and reactive and to adopt provocative attitudes in their relationships. Not everyone who expresses opposition has ODD! It's important to **decode what lies behind** oppositional behavior; there may be a number of explanations.

For instance, children (and adults, for that matter!) may adopt **oppositional behavior** in order to attract attention or to refuse to do a task (because they don't want to do it, because it doesn't make sense to them, or because they feel anxious and unable to cope with the demand, and are expressing this feeling in their own way).

For some, especially people with an Anxiety Disorder or Autism Spectrum Disorder (ASD), hypersensitivity to new instructions and transitions can translate as rigidity, obstinance or going into crisis mode. This type of attitude can be disorienting, especially when the individual's reaction is intense. It can incite feelings of anger or helplessness in those who witness it, and can lead to a reactive response and attitudes that incite conflict — resulting in escalation. Adults should act wisely and responsibly when dealing with children or young adolescents who are being oppositional, and should try to unmask the causes without inviting conflict. It's no small challenge! The **C rules** are a summary of the winning strategies for all involved: aim for **C**lear and **C**oherent instructions, **C**ommunicated in advance, with agreement on the **C**onsequences, and applied in a **C**alm and **C**onsistent way. For older adolescents and adults, it is important to develop strategies to reduce the intensity and impacts of their oppositional behavior, so their interpersonal relationships aren't overly affected .

A small proportion of young people with ADHD — primarily boys — present severe behavioral problems, called Conduct Disorder. These young people are at significantly greater risk of developing drug addiction and antisocial behavior, which can lead to legal problems. Some develop a Personality Disorder when they reach adulthood. However, this type of problem only affects a small percentage of people with ADHD. With age and maturity, behavior disorders tend

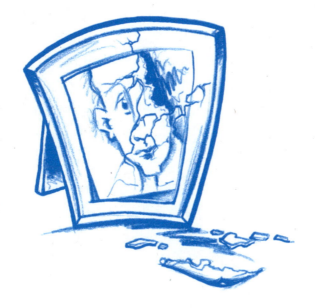

to either diminish or solidify. For persons with ADHD complicated by major behavioral problems that have led to legal difficulties, it has been shown that ADHD medication, by reducing the impulsivity associated with the condition, can also reduce the risk of recidivism. Important: **ADHD is an explanation, but not an excuse.** Taking responsibility is crucial. Thus, proper guidance, well-established instructions and a systematic application of consequences, including legal proceedings for offenses, should form an integral part of any intervention plan.

Anxiety, depression, self-esteem and self-confidence

Almost half of people affected by ADHD will develop anxious or depressive symptoms at some point in their lives. It's important to detect these problems and treat them properly. Anticipation anxiety — fear of not succeeding or of making mistakes — is often associated with ADHD and can be improved when traditional ADHD treatment helps the person experience fewer failures and regain self-confidence. One should distinguished anticipatory anxiety symptoms from standard Anxiety Disorders which include Generalized Anxiety Disorder, Panic Disorder, Obsessive-Compulsive Disorder (OCD) and Post-Traumatic Stress Disorder. The brain is unable to focus well or remain alert when it is flooded with anxiety, which can imitate the symptoms of ADHD or complicate them. It is essential to understand **what causes the brain to be distracted**.

It's like I have two hamsters running around in my head... One is going this way and that, drawn to any stimulation that attracts its attention (ADHD), and the other is stuck on its wheel, going around and around (Generalized Anxiety Disorder – GAD).

Jean, age 35

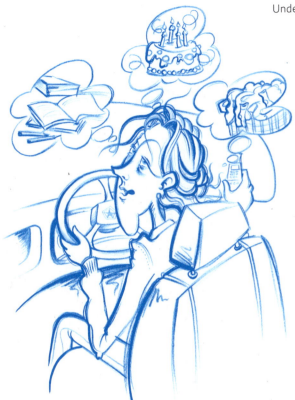

A person with ADHD would probably say "Everything!" Whatever they see, hear, perceive or think results in a getaway car of ideas speeding through their mental landscape. This mental restlessness is distinct from attentional difficulties that result from worrisome preoccupations that seize thought and trap the person in a cognitive loop that is hard to escape.

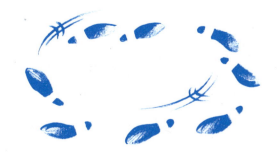

Finding the optimal level of stimulation for ADHD treatment requires a delicate balance, which can be more difficult to reach when an anxiety disorder is present. Some people suffering from associated ADHD experience an increase in pre-existing symptoms of anxiety when the dosage of a psychostimulant is too high. It is important to distinguish this phenomenon from usual side effects of these medications (see Step 5, p. 153).

Because of the impacts associated with ADHD, many who have the condition develop fragile self-esteem and a chronic sense of underachievement. Some say they feel they aren't good enough, and that their results fail to reflect their efforts. Even when they succeed, they feel like "imposters" and live in fear of one day being "found out." The sadness and angst associated with low self-esteem doesn't necessarily correspond to what could be called "Major Depressive Disorder." Even children and adolescents can be affected. It is essential to recognize this condition and to treat it adequately if it is present since depression can have serious consequences, including suicide.

Emotional hyperreactivity is often present in persons with ADHD and can sometimes be mistaken for manifestations associated with Bipolar Disorder. Persons affected with Bipolar Disorder present cyclical mood changes that are independent of events, with abrupt

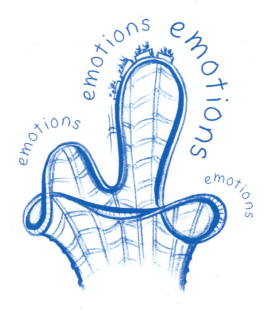

variations in energy. Hypomanic phases typically involve euphoric or irritable emotional states, punctuated by accelerated ideas with increased energy despite a diminished need for sleep. Depressive phases, on the other hand, involve sad, morose or irritable moods, associated with slowed ideas, physical and cognitive fatigue and non-restorative sleep. Keeping a mood journal can help better quantify these variations. Persons affected with Bipolar Disorder are often more sensitive to the side effects of ADHD medication, and often report discomfort in terms of mood, with feelings of feverishness and irritability. When ADHD is complicated by the coexistence of Bipolar Disorder, diagnosis and treatment requires a higher degree of expertise.

Seeking stimulation

The ADHD brain needs more stimulation to activate and self-modulate. Without quite being aware of what they're doing, some with the condition give themselves "treatment" of "homemade stimulants," like the adrenaline high from a last-minute sprint or thrill-seeking activities.

People living with ADHD present a higher risk to smoke cigarettes compared to the general population. It's not unusual to see adolescents and adults with ADHD consuming large quantities of caffeine by drinking coffee, as well as soft drinks and energy drinks. Persons with ADHD are also at a higher risk for substance abuse. They may try to calm themselves down with alcohol or cannabis and to hyperstimulate with cocaine or speed. The scientific literature is clear: these products can be toxic for the brain and are NOT recommended for treating ADHD.

Scientific studies have also shown that early medical treatment of ADHD with psychostimulants does not increase the risk of developing a substance abuse problem among young people with ADHD, and could even reduce the risk.

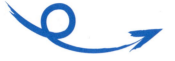

GOOD TO KNOW

ADHD is no laughing matter! Studies have shown that it increases the risk of developing or worsening many problems, such as:

- learning difficulties
- dropping out of school
- underachievement at work, frequent job changes (quitting or being fired), lower salary for equivalent education level
- anxiety
- low self-esteem
- depression
- bipolar disorder
- oppositional defiant disorder
- relationship problems, marital separation
- difficulty in adopting and maintaining a healthy lifestyle
- sleep disorders
- overuse of screens and video games
- problems with smoking, alcohol and drug use, such as cannabis or cocaine
- delinquency

- impulsive spending, financial management problems and personal bankruptcy
- psychosocial trauma
- accidental injuries, such as cuts, fractures and head injuries that require emergency room visits
- motor vehicle accidents (as a pedestrian or driver)
- unplanned pregnancies and sexually transmitted infections
- obesity
- diabetes, metabolic syndrome, high blood pressure and other cardiovascular health conditions
- difficulty in consistently taking medication and monitoring the treatment of associated chronic diseases
- reduced healthy life expectancy
- increased risk of premature death due to associated diseases, accidents or suicide

Treatment of ADHD could reduce these impacts, which underlines the importance of screening and access to resources so that every person living with ADHD enjoys a life that is less disrupted by such obstacles.

The faces of ADHD during the different stages of life

The manifestations of ADHD are similar at every age, but their intensity and their impacts on daily life are shaped by the context and modulated by the strategies implemented to compensate for them. As a person grows up, it is above all inattention, and to a lesser degree hyperactivity/impulsivity, that pushes people to seek help. Restlessness becomes less disruptive and more internalized, but it is still present, though often better channelled.

Each individual is different. Everyone has their own personality, a certain intellectual potential, a capacity to learn and different abilities and challenges. Each of us is also exposed to an environment that helps us flourish or hinders us. All these factors and many others will affect a person's outcome. Generally, a supportive environment, the absence of associated problems and an adequate IQ are elements that promote positive development for someone with ADHD.

The following tables provide a picture of the different faces ADHD can present at different ages.

Attention problems

Children...

- ○ have difficulty sustaining interest and paying attention
- ○ become scattered, move from one game to the next and leave homework aside
- ○ forget homework easily, lose things, leave things that they need at school
- ○ often become obstinate or angry when it's time to do homework, tend to avoid activities requiring sustained application or prolonged mental effort
- ○ make careless mistakes (blunders)
- ○ are easily distracted by noise (conversations, ringtones, music, etc.) and visual stimuli
- ○ have difficulty following instructions at school, in games and at home
- ○ have reading difficulties, skips words or lines, lose the thread; reading comprehension and extracting relevant information are difficult
- ○ have a hard time collecting ideas and structuring thoughts; writing texts and doing long projects can therefore be difficult

Adults...

- ▷ have the same difficulties as children, but they can become even more significant with increased complexity of tasks and less direction or supervision
- ▷ have difficulty following long conversations; this lack of attention may be interpreted by others as indifference
- ▷ miss or forget appointments or show up late
- ▷ continue to misplace things (keys, wallet, items on a shopping list, etc.)
- ▷ check and re-check, become hyperorganized with routines that may seem extremely rigid, spend a great deal of time, energy and effort to mitigate the impacts of certain symptoms (in order to isolate themselves from distracting stimuli, reduce forgetfulness and minimize the loss of objects, etc.)

Difficulties with organization

Children...

o function better under one-on-one supervision

o become disorganized when exposed to too much stimuli

o have trouble getting started, wait until the last minute, are often late

o lack order with their personal belongings at school, as well as in their bedroom

o work better with rapid feedback, as close as possible to the moment when the task is performed (but the effects are temporary and guidance must be maintained)

Adults...

▷ have difficulty getting organized in their daily lives and making long-term plans

▷ get ready and act at the last minute and are often late

▷ add tasks to their schedule as they go, thinking "I have enough time"

▷ feel the need to work on multiple projects at once

▷ have a hard time managing their paperwork and budget

▷ lack order at the office and at home

Fidgetiness

Children...

- o feel and act as though propelled by a motor: they move around a lot, move their hands, scribble, doodle, drum their fingers, wriggle in their chair, swing their feet; they run and climb all over, in inappropriate situations, at school or at home
- o get called "chatterbox" or similar names
- o often get up in the middle of a television show or a movie, during meals or during class or homework time
- o are often bumbling, go too fast, knock things over and break them or bump into things
- o lose interest easily, respond better to stimuli that changes and moves, like video games
- o write too quickly and have handwriting that's hard to read

Adults...

- ▷ are still fidgety, although this appears to attenuate with age
- ▷ fidget more discreetly by moving their hands and feet and try to control themselves by crossing their arms and legs
- ▷ have difficulty sitting still during classes, meetings, movies, and television programs
- ▷ prefer to stand rather than sit
- ▷ have difficulty relaxing or remaining calm, which is sometimes described as a nervous or anxious feeling
- ▷ are bored and sleepy when there isn't enough stimulation
- ▷ seek leisure activities and work that involve movement — immobility generates tension or anxiety
- ▷ dislike routine — they seek strong sensations in extreme sports, speed, compulsive gambling; some become video game addicts
- ▷ have difficulty engaging in calm and sedentary activities

Impulsivity

Children...

- o are disruptive and interrupt others
- o seem impatient — they want everything, right away
- o have difficulty planning future activities — "I think, therefore I act" — and rarely take the time to reflect on their actions
- o have a hard time taking into account the danger or social impact of their words and actions
- o may hurt themselves: children with ADHD are more prone than others to have accidents requiring emergency medical treatment

Adults...

- ▷ control themselves more easily than do children, but have to make an effort to slow down because they're still impulsive
- ▷ make impulsive decisions that undermine their personal and work relationships and finances and may lead to frequent relocation and job changes
- ▷ find waiting hard to tolerate
- ▷ may drive fast and impulsively, leading to higher risk of accidents in everyday life, as a driver but also as a pedestrian
- ▷ become sexually active at an early age and are at higher risk for unplanned pregnancies and sexually transmitted diseases

Emotional hyperreactivity

Children...

o feel overwhelmed by waves of emotion and often have fits of anger or crying

o are easily excitable and find it hard to calm down afterward

o blame themselves for their forgetfulness, lateness, and difficulty following instructions

o may be seen by others as mean-spirited, airheaded, or oppositional

o have low self-esteem

o frequently have the impression of not being good enough, and consequently expect failure

Adults...

▷ overreact to events and get angry easily

▷ complain of being oversensitive, frequently tearing up and feeling on edge

▷ are bored by routine

▷ have chronically low self-esteem

▷ have the impression of being inadequate, that something is wrong with them, and consequently expect failure

Interpersonal problems

Children...

- o may be seen as bossy, controlling or oppositional, which undermines relationships and friendships
- o are forgetful and error-prone
- o may be rejected by peer group due to fidgetiness and impulsiveness
- o may be more easily accepted when they clown around
- o often appear withdrawn if very inattentive

Adults...

- ▷ have more difficulty following rules if they were oppositional as children, and may seem provocative because of this
- ▷ complain often of being easily bored and seek change for the sake of change, hence the difficulty staying in relationships for a long time — difficulties maintaining stable relationships lead to higher separation and divorce rates and more partners
- ▷ have difficulty maintaining stable work — may hold more jobs for shorter periods of time and be more likely to quit or be fired

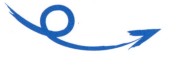

GOOD TO KNOW

Transgenerational impacts

Families with a parent or child with ADHD tend to have more tension and discipline problems. It can be hard for parents with untreated ADHD to implement and maintain organizational and emotion management strategies to help their child, because they themselves face significant challenges in these areas.

My friends tease me and call me "the tornado". I was always a "fast kid" who was constantly in motion, impulsive and talkative. I'm cheerful, friendly and very athletic. In elementary school, I succeeded in overcoming my forgetfulness and other difficulties and was able to get organized. My parents and my teachers were there to help and supervise me. High school was harder, but thanks to summer courses, I was able to make it to college. What a disaster that was! I was incapable of following lectures that lasted for three continuous hours and had to drop out after one semester. At work, my boss appreciated my dynamism, but criticized my numerous careless mistakes, my frequent lateness, and my difficulty following instructions. The result: unemployment!

My girlfriend couldn't take it anymore. She even asked me if I was interested in our relationship. The fact is, I couldn't stand long conversations. I would lose track, move around and become impatient. She was thinking about leaving me. Everything was going badly. I was completely overwhelmed and anxious and wasn't sleeping well. I saw a report on ADHD on television. It was as if they were talking about me. That decided it: I went to see my doctor. He diagnosed me with combined ADHD. Since then the treatment has been effective and has led to a remarkable change in my quality of life. It's been three years now. I've gone back to school — successfully, this time. I'll graduate soon, but the most important thing is that I have found a balance in my life, and that's incredibly precious.

Jonathan, age 25

I'm the mother of two boys whom I adore. Looking at me today, you'd never guess what I've been through. I've had ADHD since childhood, but I wasn't diagnosed until I was 16, when I almost killed myself.

I was never hyperactive. When I was little, I was called scatterbrained. I was always distracted, disorganized and very sensitive. Emotions often overwhelmed me, like a huge wave, and I would isolate myself to cry. My moods were as volatile as the weather. Because I was distracted by sounds, as well as by my own thoughts, I wasn't able to follow in class. I dropped out at the end of elementary school. By the time I was 10, I was constantly telling myself that I

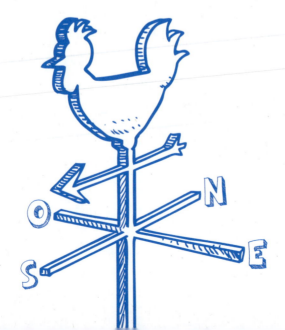

was worthless and that I wouldn't get anywhere in life. When I was 13 or 14, I started taking drugs with other kids I thought were my "friends." I quickly discovered that marijuana helped me sleep. I started using it every evening. I was laughed at and called a pothead.

Discouraged and tired of my life, I swallowed a bottle of pills. I was rushed to the emergency room. It was there that I saw a doctor who recognized my ADHD symptoms. I was given information and support, and I started medication. I also restructured my life and stopped using marijuana.

I slowly made it back to the surface. I regained confidence in myself. I found a study program that interested me. I'm doing better: I take medication and work every day to overcome the symptoms of ADHD. My son Kevin also has ADHD. I hope with all my heart that he doesn't have to follow my path and that people will not be as hard on him as they were on me when I was little.

Melanie, age 38

I run a company. I'm married and I have a five-year-old son and an eight-year-old daughter. I learned that I had ADHD when my daughter was diagnosed last year. She is a miniature copy of me. I was "the artist in the family". I was able to see things differently. In my work, having original and innovative ideas is an advantage. I'm lucky to have an entire team backing me up, because I'm still as disorganized as I was as a child.

Don't ask me to go to a movie: I can't sit still that long. I need to move, or I get wound up and feel terribly tense. Sports have always been a big part of my life.

When I was younger, it was hard to pay attention in class. Even though I was "spacey" and agitated, I would always manage to find a way to get out of things. What a clown I was! My parents and my teachers helped me. When I got to university, I rushed through my program and went straight into business. My wife helps me enormously: she's my "organizational coach". Thanks to my adaptive strategies and the support network I have around me, things are going fast, but well. As my friends would say, I'm "hard to follow."

Paul, age 43

CHECKLIST FOR STEP 1

Let's review the main points presented in this section:

> Not everyone who gets spaced out or moves around a lot has ADHD!

> There are different types of attention.

> Various factors impact our ability to self-modulate.

> The cognitive processes that allow us to concentrate for a long time and disregard distracting stimuli are those that are affected by ADHD.

> The difficulties with self-modulation associated with ADHD are manifested by symptoms of inattention and/or hyperreactivity/impulsivity sometimes associated with emotional hyperreactivity.

> The symptoms of ADHD are present in childhood and remain problematic in adulthood for the majority of sufferers.

> ADHD results in functional impacts and affects different spheres of life (personal, social, familial, conjugal, academic and/or professional).

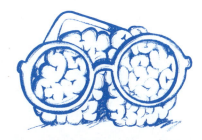

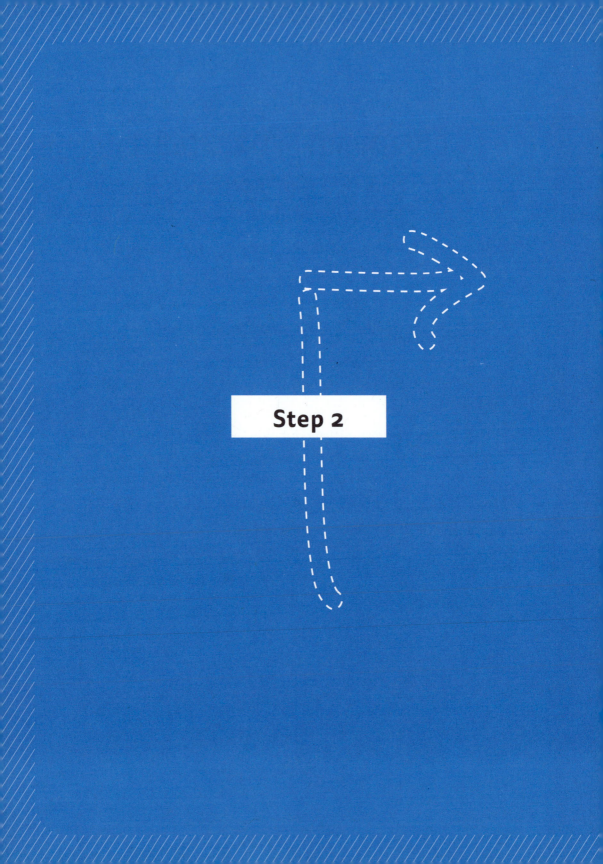

Step 2

SCIENTIFIC
STOPOVER

> **ADHD** under the magnifying glass

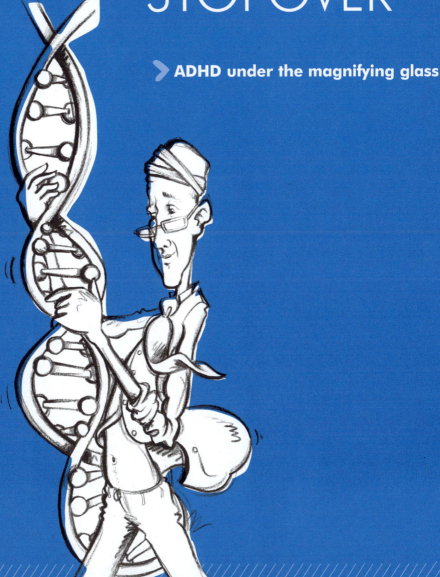

Let's make a short detour to look at what the scientific literature tells us about the genetic and environmental factors related to ADHD and the differences in brain function for people who have the condition.

Genetics

Genetic studies have shown that there is a substantial **hereditary transmission factor,** as certain genes modulate transmission of height, hair and eye color. In the majority of cases, a familial link can be found. Manifestations of ADHD can take different forms within the same family. So, a mother whose ADHD mainly manifests as inattention may have a child who does not exhibit any significant symptoms of the condition, and another child who is affected, but with predominant agitation and impulsivity. Also, for many families, the response to medication can vary from one person to another. A number of research projects are attempting to identify the genes that are involved in transmitting ADHD, but currently no genetic test exists that could clarify a diagnosis of ADHD or could predict which medication will be best tolerated or most effective.

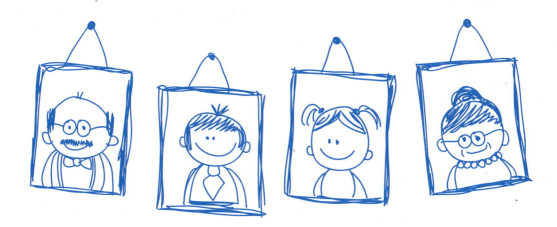

Environmental factors that should be considered

Environmental factors that cause early brain damage can also contribute to the development of ADHD. These include elements that can affect the brain's development *in utero*, such as exposure to toxins like tobacco and heavy metals (lead, for instance), as well as gestational diabetes and multiple pregnancies. Subsequent events that can "injure the brain," such as birth or early life complications (for instance, prematurity, lack of oxygen, as well as infections and head injuries), can also lead to ADHD symptoms that resemble those with a genetically modulated origin.

A brain that works differently

An orchestra conductor with no rhythm

To illustrate the impact of ADHD on cognitive functioning, Dr. Thomas Brown, an internationally renowned U.S. psychologist, compares the brain's coordinating role to that of an orchestra that can't create harmonies because the musicians are unable to synchronize. The role of the conductor is analogous to the executive functions of the brain. Any particular task is like a piece of music, and the musicians represent, for example, memory, attention, movements, ideas and emotions.

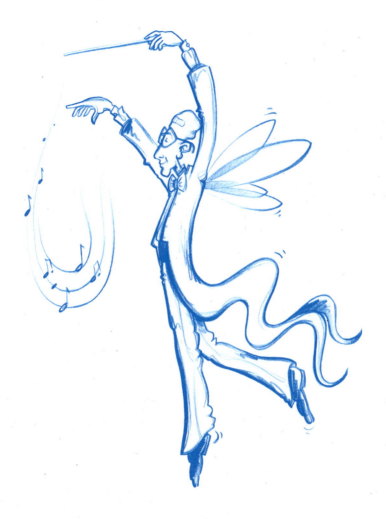

When the brain is affected by ADHD, the orchestra may still be filled with excellent musicians, but their success is undermined by the conductor, who is too drowsy, unable to keep a beat or coordinate the players. The musicians all play in their own way, following their individual rhythm and the intensity of the moment. A symphony quickly degenerates into a cacophony. In the following steps, we will

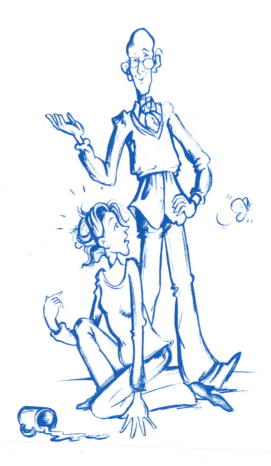

look at how adaptive strategies play the role of "psychological glasses" that help the musicians focus, despite the conductor's disorganized leadership. Similarly, medications used to treat ADHD give the conductor a "pair of biological glasses," so that they can direct the musicians effectively.

Neurons that aren't communicating properly

The flow of information in our brain related to ideas, movements, behaviors or emotions, runs through a large network of nerve cells called **neurons.** In order for one neuron to "talk" to another, it releases **neurotransmitters.** Those act like special keys that fit into a lock: the **receptor** on a neighboring neuron. This sets off a chain of biological events that induce changes that modulate the initial message: transmitting it, slowing it down or speeding it up (see *The flow of information* box, *p. 88*).

Different neurotransmitters are involved in the process of self-modulation. Studies have shown that underlying mechanisms of attention are very complex and indicate that the therapeutic effect of ADHD medications is likely linked to their capacity to support the actions of dopamine and norepinephrine in the synaptic gap. These neurotransmitters help us analyze stimuli and regulate the responses they provoke. They do this by helping to modulate attention to any novel stimuli, improving the capacity to put aside or inhibit distractors, while facilitating sustained interest and adjusting the emotional importance associated with a task. This allows us to organize our thoughts according to each project, to get started more effectively, to pass over what isn't relevant and to remain focused on what we want to achieve.

The flow of information

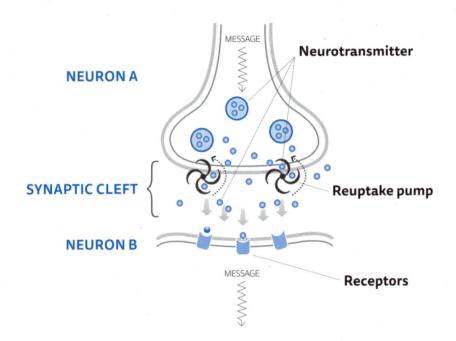

MESSAGE

Neurotransmitter

NEURON A

SYNAPTIC CLEFT

Reuptake pump

NEURON B

MESSAGE

Receptors

Information, in the form of a nerve impulse, runs through a network of nerve cells, called neurons. When it arrives at one side of the synaptic gap, the presynaptic terminal, an impulse sets off a cascade of biochemical events that induces the release of a neurotransmitter (for example, noradrenaline or dopamine) into the space between two neurons, known as the synaptic cleft. These molecules act as chemical messengers by binding to the neuron receptors – a bit like a key fitting in a lock – setting off another series of biochemical events that allows the message to circulate and be modulated. The neurotransmitters will eventually be recovered by the reuptake pump to avoid an excess of neurotransmitters in the synaptic cleft. ADHD medications act at the level of the synapse (see Step 5, p. 153, for further details).

A brain that develops and activates differently

Research protocols using brain imaging technologies allow us to compare groups of people who have ADHD with groups that don't, in order to find out whether there are anatomical or functional differences between them.

These undertakings use brain images obtained by magnetic resonance imaging and computer-assisted axial tomography — commonly called MRI and CAT scans, respectively. These images reveal slight anatomical differences. A brain affected by ADHD has a

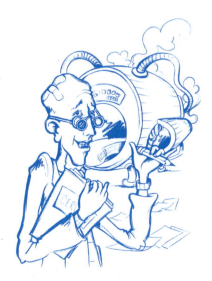

different volume in certain regions. While these differences have significant repercussions, they are so subtle that they would not necessarily be observable by examining a single affected individual. Research has found evidence of delayed development of some cortical areas in young people with ADHD, which may explain immature behavior observed in some children, adolescents and young adults with the condition. This may also explain the clinical improvement that comes with age for certain manifestations of the condition: for instance, hyperactivity and impulsivity, which often diminish in adulthood.

To examine the brain "in action," cutting-edge technologies such as functional magnetic resonance imaging (fMRI) and positron emission tomography (PET scans) are used. These complex tests reveal a different level of activation in certain areas of an ADHD-affected brain, which requires more stimulation than the brain of individuals without ADHD. It's interesting to note that motivation and ADHD medication are modulator-activators for these areas (see *Step 5*, p. 153 for more information.)

Brain imaging is useful to researchers to understand the underlying mechanisms of ADHD, but it is not recommended as a standard procedure for the clinical diagnosis or treatment of ADHD.

CHECKLIST FOR STEP 2

Let's review the main points
presented in this section:

> ADHD is a neurobiological disorder whose transmission is strongly influenced by genetics.

> Neurobiological studies reveal that individuals with ADHD may have an imbalance in the neurotransmission of dopamine and no-radrenaline, two substances that play a very important role in analyzing stimuli and modulating responses to them.

> Imaging studies show delayed maturation in the brain develop-ment of young people with ADHD and different brain function-ing in persons with ADHD. Activating certain cerebral areas requires more stimulation for persons with ADHD than it does for control groups (made up of individuals without ADHD). Motivation and ADHD medication are modulator-activators of these areas.

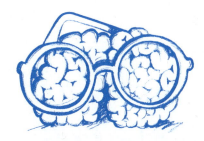

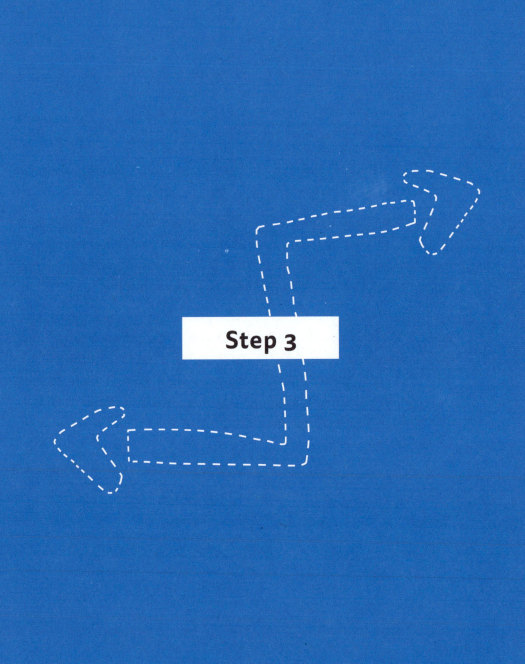

Step 3

THE DIAGNOSTIC
APPROACH

> **Everything you need to know
about the consultation process**

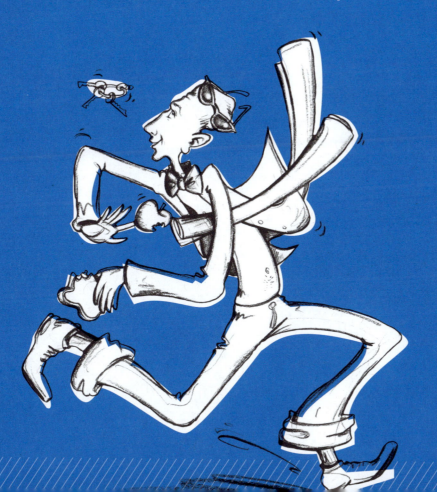

Let's explore the different paths that can lead to a diagnosis of ADHD. What prompts someone to see a doctor? What are the main steps to follow? What criteria orient clinicians in their approach?

Usually younger individuals who enter into the consultation process are guided by a parent, often as a result of problems at home or at school. Older individuals usually initiate the process themselves. Some do so because they recognize themselves in descriptions of ADHD they have read. Others do so because someone close to them, often a child, has received a diagnosis of ADHD and is getting proper treatment. They want to understand if some of their own problems stem from ADHD and, if so, to seek advice to find helpful strategies. In some cases, people see a doctor because of related problems such as anxiety, depression, relationship difficulties or substance abuse. In all cases, it's important that the clinician adopt a rigorous approach to determine whether something else is mimicking ADHD and whether actual ADHD is being aggravated by certain factors.

Who can diagnose ADHD?

The trajectory of services and access to diagnostic evaluation and therapy vary in different regions of the world. In some countries, the task of diagnostic evaluation and follow-up for ADHD is limited to medical specialists. In other regions, such as North America, a number of psychologists and general practitioners have developed expertise in the field of evaluating and monitoring ADHD. In more complex cases and when an approach in a primary care setting fails to control symptoms optimally, it may be necessary to get a consultation with a specialist to clarify the diagnosis, to find guidance or for supervision of treatment.

How the diagnostic evaluation takes place

The diagnostic process for ADHD is essentially based on clinical evaluation. It takes time and may require many sessions, often involving professionals from a range of disciplines.

In order to get the whole picture and see the matter from every angle, the clinician meets with the individual personally and also, if possible, collects information from those others (parents, teachers and, for adults, spouses). The clinician uses questionnaires to better identify symptoms associated with ADHD in childhood and to determine which manifestations are still present at the time of the consultation. Impacts associated with persisting symptoms are identified and discussed. With these symptoms in mind, the compensatory burden needs to be assessed. This includes adaptative strategies, taking into account the time and energy required for them to be effective. The results will guide intervention strategies and therapeutic approaches. It is also essential to look for related problems, since their presence can complicate both diagnosis and treatment.

The role of additional tests

There are no neuropsychological, biological or medical imaging tests that alone can confirm or disprove an ADHD diagnosis. Normally a doctor will decide to turn to these tests when there is reason to investigate the presence of other problems.

The study of executive functions in clinical research today is leading us to a better understanding of the challenges associated with ADHD. Different neuropsychological tests allow us to better evaluate some executive functions by comparing groups of individuals. However, **no single neuropsychological test can lead to or discard a diagnosis of ADHD beyond all doubt, without a clinical evaluation**. Researchers are now attempting to develop neuropsychological tests that would better characterize attentional difficulties and those related to executive functions. Experts agree that neuropsychological testing is recommended to identify specific learning disabilities and to assess IQ if a problem of this type is identified.

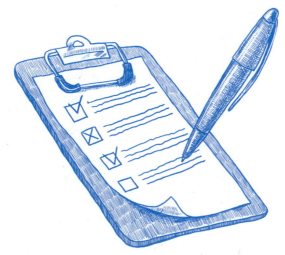

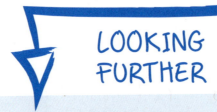

LOOKING FURTHER

Organize information-gathering

There are different questionnaires that directly target symptoms associated with ADHD. Among them, many clinicians use the SNAP-IV-26, the ASRS, the ADHD Checklist or a series of specific questionnaires devised by Conners, Brown and Barkley. Dr. Sandra Kooïj, a psychatrist working in the Netherlands, and her team developed a questionnaire specifically designed to assess adult ADHD (DIVA 5.0). The *Adult Self-Report Scale* (ASRS), helps screen adult ADHD and can also be used for older adolescents. When ADHD symptoms are identified in adulthood, it is important to determine whether some symptoms were also present in childhood. The *Weiss Symptom Record* (WSR, WSR-2) allows us to explore the presence of associated problems that could mimic or complicate ADHD. Beyond the mere presence of ADHD symptoms, it is important to measure their impacts in order to target strategies to better cope with ADHD. The *Weiss Functional Impairment Rating Scale* (WFIRS) questionnaire supports this approach by helping to identify impacts on different spheres of life from the perspective of parents (WFIRS-P) and the perspective of the affected individuals and those around them (WFIRS-S).

But, beware! Various conditions can lead to positive responses to these questionnaires. These tools are only indicators of the presence or absence of symptoms and help to quantify their intensity. They do not result in a diagnosis. Let's compare the use of these questionnaires to a thermometer used for a fever. Reading the thermometer tells you the degree of body temperature; it quantifies the fever but doesn't identify its origins. A high score on an ADHD questionnaire indicates nothing more than a high probability that the individual may suffer from the condition, but it by no means guarantees a diagnosis. Only a professional can properly assess what best explains the symptoms — hence the importance of consulting a clinician with expertise in ADHD. For instance, an anxious person can be distracted by their worries; focusing on their concerns causes them to become forgetful and makes it harder to pay attention to anything else. Anxiety tends to make an individual freeze up when facing a task; conversely an individual with ADHD who has difficulty undertaking and carrying out a task may need to feel a sense of urgency to be able to get started at the last minute. An anxious person is hypervigilant and easily startled, overly affected by ambient noise, while a person with ADHD is hypersensentive to distracting stimuli. It should be noted that tension and agitation associated with anxiety can be hard to distinguish from ADHD.

The Questionnaires section on the site attentiondeficit-info.com contains many of the questionnaires mentioned here.

ADHD criteria

To make a diagnosis of ADHD, all the following characteristics should be present, whatever the age of the person being assessed:

ADHD symptoms:

- ☒ have been present since early childhood. In adolescents and adults, one should be able to trace symptoms of inattention or hyperactivity-impulsivity before or by the age of 12

- ☒ have persisted for at least six months

- ☒ appear in at least two different settings (e.g., home, school, work)

- ☒ have led to significant functional impairment in various spheres of daily life (social, academic or professional)

- ☒ are not better explained by another psychiatric, medical or psychosocial condition and do not correspond to the normal level of development for the person's age

A minimum number of symptoms in the following list should be observable:

- ☐ 16 years or under: **AT LEAST 6 OF THE 9** symptoms of inattention and/or hyperactivity/impulsivity

- ☐ 17 years or older: **AT LEAST 5 OF THE 9** symptoms of inattention and/or hyperactivity/impulsivity

1. Inattention

The individual:

☐ has difficulty paying attention to details and makes careless mistakes

☐ has difficulty sustaining attention

☐ seems not to be listening when being spoken to directly

☐ doesn't follow instructions or finish tasks (without this being oppositional behavior)

☐ has difficulty planning and organizing work or activities

☐ avoids, postpones or reluctantly performs tasks that require sustained mental effort

☐ loses objects necessary for their work or other activities

☐ is easily distracted by external stimuli or their own thoughts

☐ frequently forgets things in daily life

2. Hyperactivity/ Impulsivity

Motor hyperactivity/The individual

☐ often fidgets with hands and feet or squirms in chair

☐ often gets up in situations where one should remain sitting

☐ runs around and climbs a lot (with increasing age: feeling of restlessness or fidgetiness)

☐ has a hard time keeping still at school, work or in recreational activities

☐ is often excited or worked up

☐ often talks too much

Impulsivity/The individual:

☐ answers questions before they are finished

☐ has difficulty waiting their turn

☐ often interrupts or intrudes upon others

Presentations of ADHD

Combined ADHD = meets criteria 1 and 2 (the most common form).
ADHD with predominant inattention = only meets criteria 1.
ADHD with predominant hyperactivity = only meets criteria 2.

Adapted from *Diagnostic and Statistical Manual of Mental Disorders*, Fifth Edition (DSM-5), American Psychiatric Association, Washington DC, 2013.

Factors that influence the expression of ADHD

The symptoms of ADHD are modulated by various factors such as the degree of stimulation, the duration of the task and the presence of distracting stimuli. Manifestations are reduced when the task is of short duration, when the person is interested, motivated and stimulated by the task or when they are less bombarded by different auditory and visual stimuli or by their own thoughts. This fluctuating performance, based on context, can complicate diagnosis and lead to misunderstandings among loved ones who don't understand the glaring and startling inconsistency.

Characteristics of situations in which ADHD symptoms are aggravated:

- ▷ tasks that require sustained attention or mental effort (school work, reports requiring synthesis, etc.)
- ▷ activities that seem uninteresting, provide no sense of novelty or immediate pleasure (paperwork, account management, etc.)
- ▷ noisy group settings (day care, school, children's parties, meetings at work, conversations with multiple people, exam room with a lot of ambient noise, etc.)

Situations in which the symptoms are less intense or minimal:

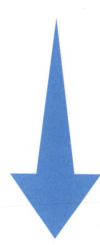

▷ tasks of short duration

▷ activities that are very interesting, that offer some immediate gain (such as video games) or that provide some novelty (such as meeting someone for the first time or having a first appointment with a doctor)

▷ situations that are closely supervised, guided or directly overseen by someone else (individual supervision or one-on-one conversation) and/or take place in an environment free of distracting external stimuli

Understanding improves actions! The following sections explore strategic interventions that allow a person living with ADHD to reach their potential.

CHECKLIST FOR STEP 3

Let's review the main points presented in this section:

> There are no neuropsychological, biological or medical imaging tests that alone can confirm or disprove an ADHD diagnosis.

> Only an authorized professional can make a diagnosis, following a rigorous evaluation, based on recognized criteria.

> The diagnostic process involves one or more meetings with the individual, and if possible, collecting of information from people around him or her (parents, teachers or, for adults, a spouse). Important points to explore include:

- The development, intensity and impact of the ADHD symptoms

- Adaptive strategies (routines, note-taking, self-correction) and the associated compensatory burden (tediousness of the task, impacts on energy and time required)

- The strengths and interests of the affected person

> An assessment of the general state of health and a check for other related problems that may mimic the presence of ADHD or complicate treatment are essential.

> A neuropsychological assessment is recommended to identify specific learning disabilities and to estimate IQ, if a problem exists in this area.

> Specific questionnaires make it possible to measure the presence and intensity of symptoms and identify their impacts.

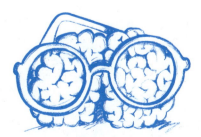

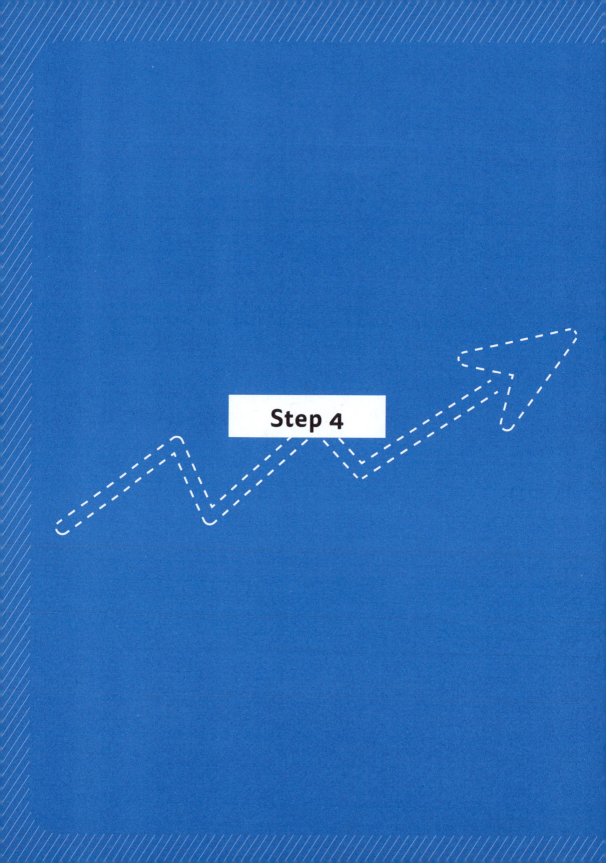

Step 4

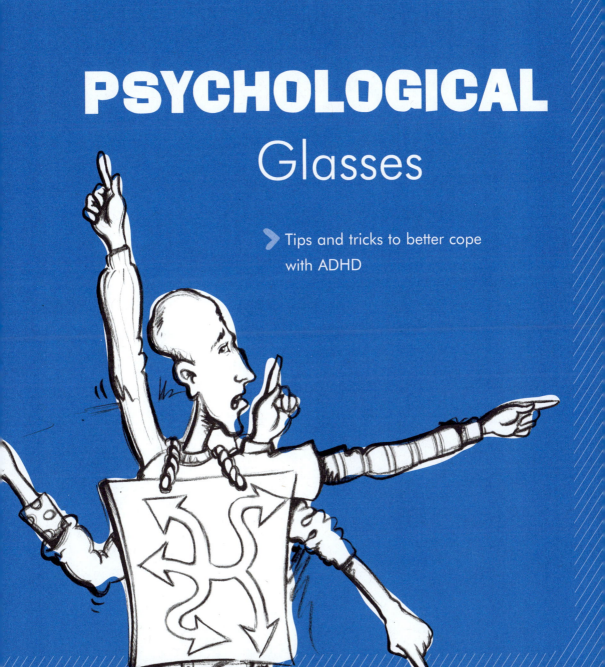

PSYCHOLOGICAL
Glasses

> Tips and tricks to better cope
with ADHD

Better controlling ADHD involves implementing adaptive mechanisms and strategies to avoid or reduce the impact of symptoms, regardless of whether the individual takes medication. Each person needs to discover the tips and tricks that work for them. To begin, let's explore the non-pharmaceutical strategies that are known to be effective.

To each their technique, to each their glasses

There's no need to wait for a diagnosis to adopt a healthy lifestyle and apply adaptive strategies that fit the symptoms that have been observed. However, it's important to consider that among individuals affected by ADHD, the very presence of the condition can cause serious difficulties when it comes to implementing and maintaining these strategies. Professional advice can help with this, even prior to diagnosis.

The first step of any ADHD treatment is to clarify the diagnosis. Labeling the problem and understanding how the brain is functioning can make it easier to implement specific therapeutic processes tailored to individual needs. For many, getting a diagnosis is a relief and leads to action. It prompts them to get mobilized, so they can incorporate solutions to better cope with ADHD. Some go through a process of mourning; others react by denying the problem. The clinician's role is to support the person and their loved ones and to help them identify the symptoms of ADHD and take stock of their repercussions on daily life, so they can target the right treatment strategies.

Learning the art of living better with ADHD

Conquering ADHD means taking charge of the therapeutic approach. ADHD explains a lot; but it doesn't excuse everything! Individuals aren't responsible for being affected with ADHD, but they are responsible for what they do with it. According to the needs identified, different resources can be suggested in the form of information and support (brochures, books, videos, Web resources, support groups).

For adequate intervention, it is important to first consider that the brain of someone affected by ADHD functions differently. It requires more stimulation to activate when sustained cognitive effort is needed. ADHD medication, as well as motivation, interest, passion and a sense of urgency, can modulate this degree of stimulation. The art of "living better with ADHD" involves identifying effective sources of stimulation to produce "just enough adrenalin" at the right moment.

The strong emotions induced by extreme sports and the stress caused by waiting until the last minute to complete a task lead to the secretion of hormones in our bodies that in turn increase the secretion of noradrenaline and dopamine — hence the expression "to be running on adrenaline". People with ADHD, especially the hyperactive-impulsive kind, often say that they are more productive and concentrate better under these conditions.

For those who function better in last-minute-sprint mode, the important thing is to learn to "procrastinate better," which means procrastinating more often but for shorter lengths of time, cutting tasks into smaller steps and making sure to set a clear deadline for each (a specific date and time). This approach transforms a long hike into a series of short, urgent sprints, resulting in a higher number of effective work periods.

Learn to procrastinate better

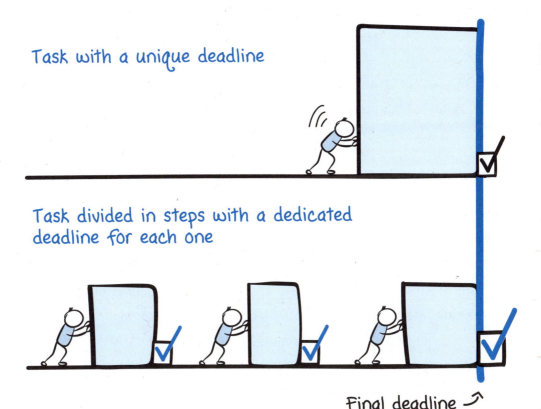

Task with a unique deadline

Task divided in steps with a dedicated deadline for each one

Final deadline ⤴

A brain with ADHD spends more time and energy pushing distracting stimuli to the side and organizing ideas, information and tasks. The process can be exhausting! It's important to guide the individual and their loved ones in implementing and maintaining specific adaptive strategies. These strategies will allow them to establish routines and to manage their time and environment differently in their personal, family, social, academic and professional lives, while taking into account their strengths and challenges.

A brain with ADHD expends a lot of effort trying to concentrate and struggling to modulate movements. Physical activity can improve wakefulness and is a precious ally in improving the ability to modulate. To be more attentive, an individual with ADHD has to "fidget to better concentrate" — but without disturbing others! It's a daily struggle to channel restlessness without bothering people nearby, and to succeed in taking planned breaks to avoid running out of steam for a task.

Incorporating healthy practices

Many conditions can modulate the intensity of ADHD symptoms. It is important to identify and reduce the impact of associated problems that affect energy levels and cognitive effectiveness. These may include an overload of work, a turbulent emotional life, absence of routine, poor health practices and toxic substance use. To limit the impact of ADHD in daily life, it's essential to adopt healthy habits and techniques for managing time and organizing tasks. Developing and maintaining a **healthy lifestyle** helps to control the symptoms of ADHD. It's a good idea for everyone to **get enough sleep**, take the time to **eat well**, take breaks to **rest** and relax, take **pleasure** in life, **exercise regularly** and **aim for a good balance** between work and pleasure.

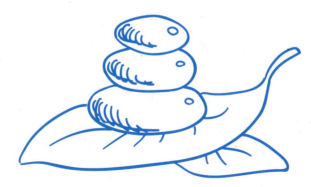

Frank is my big brother. Like our father and grandmother, we came into the world with ADHD. Dad had to take medication, but Grandma never tried it. We've found lots of tricks and tips to help overcome ADHD symptoms. To decrease the number of things I lose, my solution is to really take note of where I put my things and to adopt the principle of "everything has its place". I find that I waste less time and that there are fewer things that I need that are "temporarily misplaced". For my brother Frank, the opposite is true. He is incapable of such discipline for more than a few days and he remains disorganized. So he decided to supply himself with several copies of "essential" things. He has six sets of keys, four hammers, and I don't know how many pairs of sunglasses. That way he always has at hand what he needs until he finds the others.

Marie-Julie, age 29

I am a salesperson. In my work, I travel from one client to another, which works very well with my need for movement. I miss meetings much less often since I started managing my schedule with my electronic personal planner. I earn a good living, but I can easily waste $1,000 on parking fines. It's the classic story. I park in front of my client's store, I put money in the parking meter, and I go in. Then I lose track of time. When I have finished, the parking officer has already put a ticket on my windshield. I take the ticket and stick it some place without thinking and promptly forget about it. Weeks later, I receive a notice of late payment, including additional fines. When I learned that I had ADHD, I suddenly understood a lot of things! So I started implementing other strategies. Now, I program my electronic planner so that the alarm sounds five minutes before the time expires on my parking meter. That way I have time to wind up my visit and leave, or to return to the parking meter to put more change to cover the time that I need. With these strategies in place, I've clearly improved my quality of life and I'm doing better.

Nathalie, age 34

PRACTICAL TIPS AND TRICKS FOR DEALING WITH ADHD FROM DAY TO DAY

Let's look at a number of tips and tricks that have helped many individuals living with ADHD. Choose the ones that suit you best, and put them into practice right away!

Tips

- ➔ Check off the tricks that you are already using.
- ➔ Underline those that you would like to implement.
- ➔ Cross out those that don't work for you.
- ➔ Use those that help as much as you can.
- ➔ Be persistent and, above all, inventive, and don't hesitate to adapt them according to your specific needs.
- ➔ **Explore, and remember that everyone is unique!**
  Your solution may be different from someone else's.

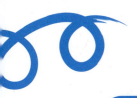

ORGANIZE YOUR TIME

Make time concrete

☐ Use your watch, an hourglass or an alarm clock to see time pass.

☐ Use a timer (that makes a noise or vibrates) as a reminder to start, finish or change tasks. Most cell phones and electronic planners have this feature.

Manage time and ideas

☐ Create a routine. By following an established order for the day, there is less risk of forgetting things.

☐ Make schedules and organizational tables, establish priorities for goals (first by their importance, then by their urgency) and set a strict deadline for each step.

☐ At work, create time blocks by theme or by type of task. For example:

➡ managing phone calls and email

➡ paperwork

➡ planning of ongoing and future work

➡ ongoing projects and tasks to complete

☐ Use the beginning or end of the day — when there are fewer people around, and therefore fewer interruptions — to do demanding work that requires more concentration.

☐ Take notes.

☐ Find a reminder system — either a notebook or a planner — rather than taking notes on slips of paper that are easy to lose.

☐ Use a personal planner:

➡ choose between a paper version and an electronic version

➡ choose a format small enough to carry with you but big enough to contain everything you need to write down

➡ keep the planner handy; decide on a place to keep it, such as next to the phone

➡ take it with you — put a note by the door if you tend to forget it

➡ write down the normal things, but also the "brilliant ideas to remember" that occur to you during the day

➡ use the planner to make a "to do" list that is color- and number-coded by priority

➡ get into the habit of consulting your planner at the beginning of the day

➡ give yourself the time to plan the day

☐ Make lists.

☐ Put written memos in strategic places, where they will be useful. Post-it® Notes are the big favorites for this.

☐ Leave yourself reminder messages on your voice mail, by text or email.

☐ Avoid scattered efforts and limit procrastination.

◻ Beware of the tendency to think "as long as I'm here..." or to plan too many tasks than is humanly possible to complete. Here are some questions to ask yourself:

➡ What are my priorities right now?

➡ Do I have a tendency to fill up my time by adding things to do and then being late?

➡ Are there too many things to do for the time available?

➡ Is the list of things to do getting longer?

◻ Avoid waiting until the last minute to do tasks. A brain with ADHD is like a sprinter; when facing a marathon, you should adapt by procrastinating better (see p. 111). So:

➡ determine priorities, first by their importance, then by their urgency

➡ estimate the amount of time needed and decide the appropriate time slot

➡ break down big tasks into small steps

➡ give yourself reasonable deadlines for each step, and respect them

➡ do one step at a time

➡ reward yourself for completing each step, not just when the task is done

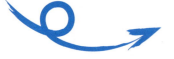

GOOD TO KNOW

Learn to adapt adaptive techniques

Using memos, personal planners and lists is useful for everyone. Russell Barkley, an internationally renowned U.S. psychologist, emphasizes the necessity of using adaptive techniques at the right time and place where they will be most useful. For example, it is more effective to place a reminder to call someone next to the telephone. Similarly, a reminder to buy milk on the way home from work won't be very handy posted on the refrigerator door, but would be much more helpful on the dashboard of your car.

ORGANIZING SPACE

Everything in its place and a place for everything!

☐ Use well-defined, transparent and clearly identified storage systems: baskets, drawers, files.

☐ Select vertical storage systems, such as upright folders containing documents, rather than horizontal systems, such as piles of documents where only the top one is visible.

- [ ] Put high-priority items and things you don't want to forget, such as paperwork you need to pay bills or documents for meetings, where you will see them.
- [ ] Use color codes (for example, red for high priorities).
- [ ] Put labels that list the contents on closed containers.
- [ ] Avoid cluttered environments.

Manage paperwork

- [ ] Avoid leaving piles of paperwork around.
- [ ] Eliminate the "to do some day" piles.
- [ ] Follow the OHIO principle: "Only Handle It Once." Take care of paperwork immediately, then send it, file it or throw it away.

Reduce time lost looking for things

- [ ] Take the time to notice where you put things.
- [ ] Decide on specific places to store important objects.
- [ ] Procure duplicate materials and equipment you need for work.
- [ ] Put identification labels on personal items. They will be easier to identify, for example, in the lost-and-found box.

REDUCE SOURCES OF DISTRACTION

Create good working conditions

☐ Find out what the best working conditions are for you:

➡ In silence or with music?

➡ Sitting, standing, while scribbling or while walking?

➡ Alone or with other people?

➡ In a calm place, removed from the center of activity?

➡ Doing a single job or running several projects at the same time?

Reduce noise distractions

☐ Use earplugs, headphones or other noise protectors .

☐ Mask sounds with background music.

☐ Isolate yourself by closing the door.

Reduce visual distractions

☐ Put away objects that are not needed in your work area.

☐ Avoid "inviting" stimuli such as a window, the television, the computer and the smartphone.

☐ Sit in front of your task or the person you are addressing while turning your back on distractions.

☐ Minimize message alerts and notifications.

Reduce internal distractions

☐ Write down ideas that come to mind so that you can come back to them later.

☐ In class or at meetings, put your ideas on paper rather than interrupting others.

☐ For tasks that you tend to space out on, take breaks to avoid losing the thread and set an alarm (with a sound or vibrating signal) to verify if you are still working on the appropriate task at that moment.

MANAGE THE FIDGETS!

In your leisure time

☐ Channel the need to move into sports activities. An active brain works better!

☐ Incorporate action and movement in your activities.

At work and in class

☐ Take breaks to loosen up.

☐ Play with an object, move discretely (for example, toes, abdominal muscles), draw, write or scribble to help channel fidgetiness when you need to remain seated.

☐ Avoid playing with noisy objects that could disturb the people around you.

IMPROVE YOUR MONEY MANAGEMENT

Managing your budget

☐ Plan expenditures in advance.

☐ Set a budget and follow it.

☐ Withdraw money from your account only once a week.

☐ Conduct transactions in cash only to reduce impulse buying.

Managing accounts

☐ Minimize the number of accounts and credit cards to manage.

☐ Take care of bills immediately:

➡ send payments as soon as the bill is received

➡ use postdated checks or make payments online

➡ make automatic payments using preauthorized payment systems

☐ Don't let receipts pile up: file them or throw them out. Remember the OHIO principle: "Only Handle It Once." (see p. 121)

CONTROL YOUR IMPULSIVITY

Reduce impulse buying

☐ Ask yourself: "Do I really need this?"

☐ Ask yourself: "Can I afford this?"

☐ Wait and come back another day for unplanned purchases.

☐ Use cash rather than bank cards or credit cards.

☐ Minimize temptations:

➡ decide how much money you can spend each week, make one withdrawal, and limit your spending to this amount

➡ avoid hanging out in stores

➡ make a shopping list before going to the store and stick to it

➡ check prices by telephone rather than at the store, be careful when you shop online...

Improve your personal relationships

☐ Try to interrupt less often.

☐ Consciously take a step back before talking or taking action, to determine the impact of your words or actions.

☐ Conquer your emotions and hyperreactivity.

☐ Go elsewhere instead of blowing up. Give yourself a time-out.

☐ Use humor to defuse tense situations.

Improve your driving

☐ Watch your speed.

☐ Use the cruise control.

☐ Respect speed limits and other traffic signs.

☐ Keep your distance.

☐ Ask your passengers not to distract you while you are driving.

☐ Avoid doing other things while driving (and never use your smartphone!).

SIMPLIFY YOUR LIFE

Delegate tasks when possible

☐ Distribute responsibility for household tasks fairly (you'll find easy-to-use tables on pp. 130-139).

☐ Hire professionals when needed for:

➡ housework

➡ maintenance of the exterior of the house

➡ tutoring or homework supervision

➡ accounting

Let others know that you have ADHD. They can help you by:

☐ Making sure that you are paying attention by creating more contact:

➡ visually (looking you in the eyes)

➡ with sound (for example, saying your name)

➡ physically (for example, gently touching your arm)

☐ Using short sentences when talking to you

☐ Sending you messages by text or email — rather than verbally (for example, by telephone)

What are the sources of stress in your life?

The brain becomes overloaded if it has to deal with intense emotions. The following questionnaire will help you determine the sources of stress in your life. Check each of the elements that contribute to your stress. Then you can use the following steps to resolve the problem:

1. First, realize that there is a problem!
2. Identify the problem and define its characteristics.
3. Make a list of imaginable solutions, from the most frivolous to the most reasonable.
4. Evaluate the pros and cons of the solutions.
5. Choose one solution.
6. Apply the selected solution.
7. Evaluate the impact of the solution.
8. Repeat as needed.

Personal factors

- [ ] Tardiness or the feeling of always arriving at the last minute
- [ ] Chronic organizational problems
- [ ] Poor self-esteem
- [ ] Fragility in terms of managing emotions

Health

- [ ] Chronic health problems
- [ ] Chronic pain
- [ ] Problems related to eating habits
- [ ] Irregular hours or lack of sleep
- [ ] Fatigue
- [ ] Lack of time for physical exercise
- [ ] Drug or alcohol problems

Finances

- [ ] Managing paperwork
- [ ] Planning a budget
- [ ] Following a budget
- [ ] Debt
- [ ] Lack of a financial cushion
- [ ] Forms (for example, tax forms)

Family

- ☐ Crisis situations (for example: death or divorce)
- ☐ Marital problems
- ☐ Supervising and raising children
- ☐ Children's challenging behaviors
- ☐ Time spent as "chauffeur" for the children
- ☐ Family member with health problems

School

- ☐ Learning difficulties
- ☐ Limited network of friends at school
- ☐ Interpersonal conflicts at school
- ☐ Failures (past or anticipated)
- ☐ Indecision about program or career orientation
- ☐ Difficulty finding balance between studies and other aspects of life

Work

- ☐ Questions concerning career orientation
- ☐ Problems at work
- ☐ Dissatisfaction with work
- ☐ Interpersonal conflicts at work
- ☐ Overbooked schedule
- ☐ Job loss
- ☐ Difficulty finding balance between work and other aspects of life

TIPS AND TRICKS FOR BETTER SHARING OF RESPONSIBILITIES

The distribution of household tasks can be a source of stress and conflict for many couples. The problem is often more bothersome in families in which one of the adults has ADHD. To simplify household organization, use a list of household chores such as the one on the following pages and proceed as follows:

Instructions

➡ Make as many copies of the list as there are people involved in doing the work, plus one.

➡ Each person completes the list.

➡ Discuss the distribution of tasks.

➡ Use the last copy of the list to record the consensus reached.

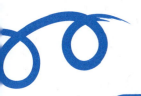

INDOOR MAINTENANCE

	How often	Person(s) responsible	Degree of satisfaction (from 0/10 to 10/10)
Entrance			
Put things away			
Dust			
Vacuum			
Wash the floor			
Living room			
Put things away			
Dust			
Vacuum			
Wash the floor			
Kitchen and dining room			
Clean the kitchen after meals			
Do dishes			
Put dishes away			
Put things away			
Dust			
Vacuum			
Wash the floor			
Clean the stove			
Clean the toaster and the microwave			
Clean the refrigerator			
Clean the oven			
Take out the garbage			

	How often	Person(s) responsible	Degree of satisfaction (from 0/10 to 10/10)
Master bedroom			
Make the bed			
Put away clothes and other items			
Dust			
Vacuum			
Wash the floor			
Children's bedroom(s)			
Make the bed			
Put away clothes and other items			
Dust			
Vacuum			
Wash the floor			
Basement			
Put things away			
Dust			
Vacuum			
Wash the floor			
Office			
Put things away			
Dust			
Vacuum			
Wash the floor			

	How often	Person(s) responsible	Degree of satisfaction (from 0/10 to 10/10)
Bathroom(s)			
Clean the sink			
Clean the counter			
Polish the mirror			
Scrub the toilet			
Clean the bathtub			
Clean the shower			
Put things away			
Dust			
Vacuum			
Wash the floor			
Other rooms			
Put things away			
Dust			
Vacuum			
Wash the floor and/or carpet			
Water the plants			
Take out the garbage			
Wash the windows			
Organize cabinets and closets			
Organize the garage			
Plan purchases of household products			
Supervise and pay a cleaning service or other household help			

LAUNDRY

	How often	Person(s) responsible	Degree of satisfaction (from 0/10 to 10/10)
Gather dirty clothes			
Wash dirty clothes			
Fold clean clothes			
Iron			
Put away clean clothes			
Wash towels			
Wash bed linens			
Laundromat / dry-clean (drop off and pick up)			

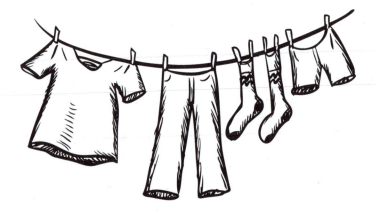

GENERAL UPKEEP

	How often	Person(s) responsible	Degree of satisfaction (from 0/10 to 10/10)
Paint			
Carpentry			
Minor repairs			
Make a plan, buy items needed to do the work			
Supervise and pay for contracted work			
Change light bulbs and smoke-alarm batteries			

OUTDOOR MAINTENANCE

	How often	Person(s) responsible	Degree of satisfaction (from 0/10 to 10/10)
Mow the lawn			
Fertilize the lawn			
Plant			
Prune trees and bushes			
Regular cleaning of patio furniture			
Pool maintenance			

	How often	Person(s) responsible	Degree of satisfaction (from 0/10 to 10/10)
Rake leaves in the fall			
Winterize (house and yard)			
Shovel snow			
Snow removal			
Spring clean-up of yard			
Maintenance of equipment, tools, supply of cleaning and gardening products			
Supervise and pay for contracted work			

FOOD

	How often	Person(s) responsible	Degree of satisfaction (from 0/10 to 10/10)
Plan meals			
Grocery shopping			
Prepare meals			
Prepare lunches			
Set the table and serve			
Manage provisions (staples, perishable items, etc.)			

CHILDREN

	How often	Person(s) responsible	Degree of satisfaction (from 0/10 to 10/10)
Care (diapers, baths, breastfeeding/meals, etc.)			
Discipline (establish and apply rules)			
Wake-up routine			
Prepare for school or daycare			
Transportation (school, daycare, sports, activities)			
Plan meals eaten away from home			
Help with homework			
Bedtime routine			
Meet with teachers			
Appointments (doctor, dentist, hairdresser, etc.)			
Special activities at school or daycare			
Attend sports or school activities			
Plan purchases (clothing, school supplies, etc.)			

	How often	Person(s) responsible	Degree of satisfaction (from 0/10 to 10/10)
Parties and birthdays (invitations, gifts, etc.)			
Arrange for babysitters			
Registrations (school, daycare, sports, recreational activities, etc.)			
Supervise and pay nanny			
Being absent from work (for example, when a child is sick)			

FINANCES

	How often	Person(s) responsible	Degree of satisfaction (from 0/10 to 10/10)
Plan the budget			
Pay bills and manage accounts			
Plan fixed expenses			
Plan purchases			
Shop for household essentials			
Complete tax forms			
Shop for mortgage, insurance, etc.			

CAR

	How often	Person(s) responsible	Degree of satisfaction (from 0/10 to 10/10)
Fill the gas tank, or charge the car			
Check the level of oil, windshield fluid, antifreeze, lubricants, tire pressure, etc.			
Change the oil			
Wash the car			
Plan and keep maintenance and repair appointments at the garage			

PETS

	How often	Person(s) responsible	Degree of satisfaction (from 0/10 to 10/10)
Feed			
Take out or walk the dog			
Change the litter box, clean cages, pick up after the dog in the yard			
Grooming, baths, nail trimming, etc.			
Train			
Visits to veterinarian			
Plan for pet sitters or boarding when out of town			

Play to your strengths

Studies in neuropsychology have shown that individuals living with ADHD have a different way of thinking and are good at finding innovative solutions. The key to success lies in the capacity to "tame" ADHD so this creativity can be expressed and put to use. Throughout history, persons with ADHD have helped enrich society with their innovative spirit and their creativity in diverse areas: the arts, science, business and sports, to name just a few!

Here is a list of certain strengths that individuals with ADHD report having, as cited by psychologist Kathleen Nadeau in her book *Adventures in Fast Forward*.[1]

▷ Good at finding innovative solutions

▷ Good in crisis situations (action-reaction)

▷ Don't stay angry for long

▷ Energetic

▷ Enthusiastic

▷ Able to improvise

▷ Very verbal

▷ Spontaneous

▷ Creative

▷ Exciting

▷ Good company

1. NADEAU, K.G. *Adventures in Fast Forward: Life, Love, and Work for the ADD Adult*, New York, Brunner/Mazel, 1996.

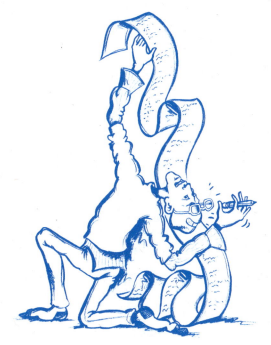

Surround yourself with the right people

Surrounding yourself with people who recognize your assets and help you to develop and blossom is a healthy strategy for everyone, with or without ADHD. It's important to find our strengths, to appreciate them and put them to use as we mature and grow, while facing our own challenges. Dr. Edward Hallowell — a psychiatrist who has ADHD himself — emphasizes in his texts and talks how important it is for people with ADHD to have helpful and encouraging people around them. Dr. Anthony Rostain, a psychiatrist, researcher and author, stresses that it is important for individuals with ADHD to identify their sources of motivation and to channel them, since **motivation** is a major factor in their ability to take action and apply effective strategies to realize their full potential.

Know how to ask for help

Support groups

Getting support from peers with similar challenges can help to de-mystify ADHD. It's also a means to find tools and break out of isola-tion. You can access an exhaustive list of support groups on the website attentiondeficit-info.com, under the ADHD section. You'll also find a number of tips and tricks, tools, reading suggestions, videos and web resources on this site.

Specialized professional help

Treating ADHD and associated problems often requires a multimo-dal approach. For instance, a **psychologist** or another specialized professional may be consulted for specific psychotherapies; a **speech language therapist** may work on learning disabilities; a **psychoeducator** can assess psychosocial adjustment and adaptive abilities; a **specialized educator** may assist with tips and tricks to better guide parents or teachers of kids with ADHD and also adults struggling with their own ADHD; an **occupational therapist** may provide assistance to develop adaptative strategies for ADHD-related problems and specially aid in cases of associated motor diffi-culties; a **social worker** may help deal with social or family problems; a **vocational counselor** could help choose an appropriate school program or career; a **financial consultant** may be useful for man-aging money or reducing debt. Some professionals also offer "orga-nizational coaching," a support service to implement and maintain specific adaptive strategies for ADHD. Unfortunately, specialized ADHD resources are still scarce in many regions today and are in need of development.

Specific psychotherapies

Studies have shown that cognitive-behavioral, mindfulness and dialectical behavior therapies have positive results, not only in reducing the impact of the classic symptoms of ADHD, but in improving emotion management and reducing impulsivity. Generally, these approaches involve strategies to help people learn more about themselves, channel their strengths and implement and maintain adaptive strategies in order to function better. Psychotherapy can also improve self-esteem and interpersonal relationships. The psychotherapist can guide a patient through periods of crisis by teaching emotion management and problem-solving tools.

For a person with ADHD, it is essential to choose structured approaches with a specific objective. The therapeutic process may be adapted in certain ways, for instance, so that the individual can take notes or record what is discussed. These sessions may be done individually, as a couple or with the family.

Another option is to work with a personal coach who provides support, somewhat like parents do for their children or an executive secretary does for the head of a company. Since there is no formal training required to become an "ADHD coach," beware of self-declared, off-the-cuff coaches. Sometimes, a friend or family member may act as a coach. Such a dynamic can be very useful, but can also become a source of tension. A clarification of roles and good mutual understanding are essential to making it work.

School support

In some countries, specific adaptative and assistance measures may be offered for students with ADHD (with or without a learning disability) who present difficulties that affect their learning or their ability to demonstrate their knowledge during exams. In order to implement a specific intervention plan in Canada a diagnosis certificate must be filled out by a professional who specifies the chronic nature of the symptoms, their impact on learning and the need for assistance measures at school. The specific measures are then determined and implemented by the school to help the student compensate for the impacts of ADHD symptoms. Note that a person living with ADHD shouldn't need to present a co-occurring learning disability to have access to these resources, which include technological aids.

Here are some assistance measures that can help support students with ADHD and help them succeed. These strategies can also be used to support individuals with ADHD in other areas of life: for instance, in the professional sphere.

▷ Permitting movement (like squeezing a stress ball, using a rolling chair, getting up, stretching, going for a walk), which prolongs the ability to maintain focus and channels restlessness.

▷ Limit the sources of distraction:

- In class, sit in a seat facing the teacher, avoid being too close to disruptive stimuli (a window or a noisy student).
- Study and write exams in a calm and quiet room.
- During study periods, limit access to smartphones (Internet and social media); wearing earplugs or noise protectors while studying and during exams helps certain students concentrate better by blocking out surrounding noise.

▷ Allocate extra time during exams so the student can adequately read the instructions, answer questions and review the answers to check for inattention errors. This also reduces the impact of periods of distraction.

▷ Allow adapting of the assessment process in order to reduce the impacts of ADHD and related problems. For instance, if ADHD and dyslexia are both present, exam questions could be read aloud.

▷ Provide access to adapted learning assistance (homework help, task supervision) and educational support to help establish healthy habits, routines and management strategies.

- Time management: plan out the day and note the time of classes and due dates for homework and exams; make a detailed schedule. For older students, an electronic planner and alarms can be used to organize tasks.
- Space management: lay out a work area with limited sources of distraction; use color coding and a filing system that makes it easy to see tasks and work to submit.
- Stress management to better modulate performance anxiety. The free application HealthMinds is handy and can be downloaded at http://healthymindsapp.ca/index.php.

▷ Provide guidance in the form of mentoring or tutoring.

▷ Providing assistance with note-taking can facilitate tasks for students who have difficulties following along and writing while listening to the teacher.

- Provide class notes in advance.
- Use a note-taker.
- Utilize a smart pen that can record what's said in class and take notes simultaneously.

▷ Permit the use of electonic assistance tools and specialized software.

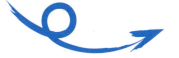

GOOD TO KNOW /////////////

Electronic assistance tools and specialized software

Writing on a computer makes it possible to create a draft that's easier to correct and structure effectively, and that can be reworked and reviewed more quickly to create a polished text. It also reduces the time spent on self-correction and cuts the number of occasions that the person has to manually transcribe or recopy the text. For homework and exams, specialized assistance software (mind mapping support, correction aids, word prediction and speech synthesis, the latter making "careless mistakes" audible) can help students notice errors and correct them. Using these valuable tools allows students to be evaluated more accurately. This type of assistance is helpful for individuals with ADHD, regardless of whether they have a verbal or written language disorder.

Allowing this kind of software to be used for writing tasks or during exams helps shift the focus to what's essential: reading well and understanding the instructions, getting started, finding ideas, building structure and following lines of thought. This allows students to organize the text, construct clear phrases that present a thought, write a coherent text using the ideas specified in the instructions and correct their work before submitting it.

A detour into "alternative" approaches

Some studies suggest that a diet rich in omega-3s of seafood origin could improve the functioning of persons with ADHD or learning disabilities and mild mood disorders, and could enhance cardio-vascular health in general.

European studies have shown that the symptoms of Restless Legs Syndrome (which can sometimes resemble the fidgetiness described by hyperactive persons) can sometimes be reduced with iron supplements when the person lacks iron, which is indicated by low ferritin levels in the blood.

More and more studies are focusing on sleep disorders associated with ADHD, and some research has shown an interesting effect from the occasional use of melatonin to "reset the body clock." However, no research has been published on its long-term (over many months) use.

Until now, research with comparitive groups hasn't shown that cognitive training and neurofeedback programs are significantly effective for treating ADHD symptoms. Experts recommend caution when considering these techniques. Those who decide to try one of these options should consider the approach as a sort of scientific study, with themselves as the sole subject. Remember: an effective approach for one person will not necessarily work for most people.

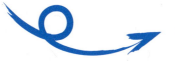 GOOD TO KNOW /////////////

Beware of charlatans!

Before undertaking any new treatment, whether it be medication, a so-called "natural product" or a special intervention technique, it's crucial to ensure that the treatment has been tested and has received official approval from a credible scientific body.

All too often we see ads with people personally endorsing the merits of some product: "It really works!" they claim. But without evidence of a significant effect on a large number of people, this type of claim can't be considered scientifically valid.

When doing your research, beware of scams and sensationalism. Be critical and approach data like a scientist. For example, when reading an advertisement or watching a commercial for a new "revolutionary" treatment, it is best to ask questions like:

- Is the source credible?
- Does the data come from studies?
- Are the theories supported by scientific evidence or are they simply one person's ideas?
- Does the treatment offer an innovative therapeutic approach?
- Has the treatment been tested on large groups of affected people? Is it safe?
- Has the treatment been shown to be effective in comparison with standard treatments and/or a placebo? Is it better tolerated?
- How much does the treatment cost? Calculate the cost, taking into consideration on the one hand the side effects and the price, and on the other, the beneficial effects.

CHECKLIST FOR STEP 4

Let's review the main points
presented in this section:

> It's essential to know what ADHD is and understand it in order to develop adaptive strategies (psychological glasses) that help reduce the impact of ADHD symptoms.

> Tips and tricks for living with ADHD include: adopting healthy lifestyle habits, taking care of oneself, taking into account factors that influence one's attention, and implementing strategies for managing time, space and emotions. These so-called "universal" strategies can help anyone with attention, hyperactivity and impulsivity difficulties, whether they are diagnosed with ADHD or not.

> Access to a support group is often beneficial.

> Psychotherapy can be helpful in many cases, as can meditation or mindfulness practice.

> Specific adaptive measures may be useful in school and at work, for instance.

It's important to consider not only the efficacy of these strategies but also the associated costs in terms of additional time and energy. When ADHD symptoms remain disabling or the compensatory burden is heavy, it's time to consider the use of medication ("biological glasses"). To each their own glasses!

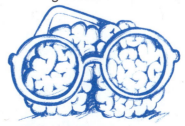

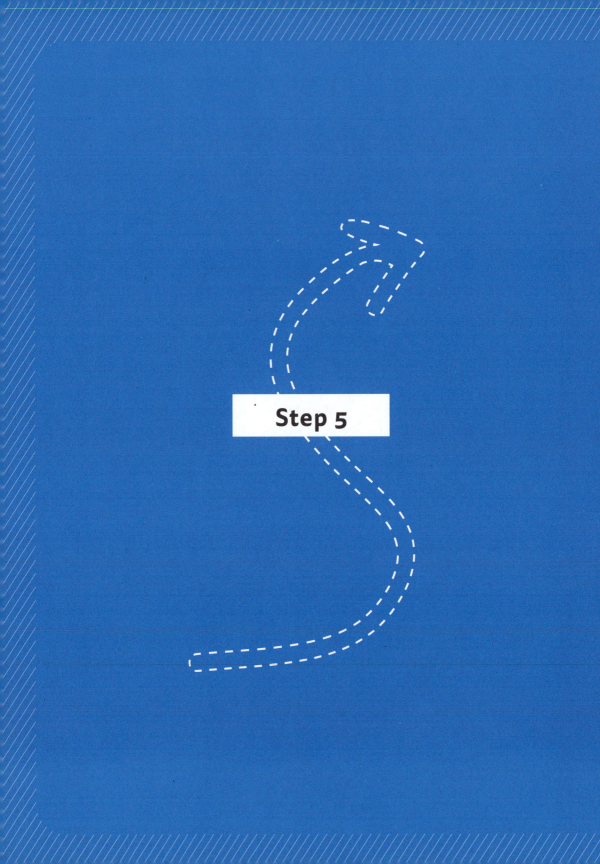

Step 5

BIOLOGICAL
Glasses

> **Pharmacological treatments: Finding your way**

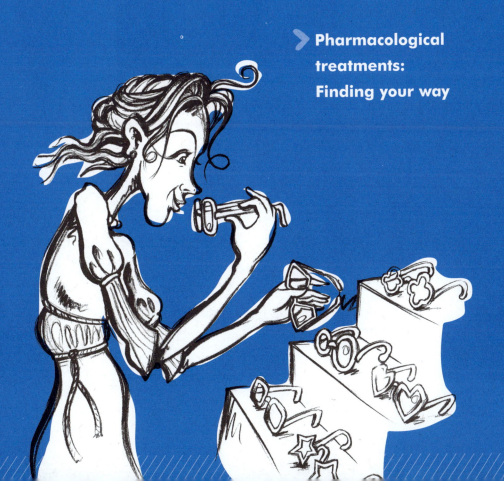

Let's complete our journey by looking at the role of medication as a strategy for living better with ADHD. It's essential to understand the basics of this subject and have a realistic sense of the possible pitfalls when taking on a pharmacological treatment.

ADHD medication: how, why, for whom?

The importance of knowing and understanding

Knowing and understanding: two steps that form an integral part of ADHD treatment. For many, they lead to a feeling of relief and hope—sometimes tinged with regret for not having identified what's happening earlier, particularly if the diagnosis comes later in life. Clarifying the diagnosis, recognizing the impacts of symptoms, understanding how ADHD influences brain functioning and learning practical tips and tricks to better cope are the first steps in the therapeutic approach.

But what factors might lead someone to consider a pharmacological treatment for ADHD? Primarily, it's important to take care of your brain to give it every chance of functioning properly. This starts with adopting healthy lifestyle practices and an attitude of self-kindness, fostering a habit of mindfulness and implementing the adaptive strategies described in the section on "psychological glasses." Clarifying the diagnosis allows for a more thorough therapeutic approach using specific targeted interventions like setting up adaptive measures at school or work. It can also lead to options for medication that's proven to be effective for treating ADHD. Identifying which factors are inherent to ADHD and which might complicate its expression, the impacts of symptoms and the moments they manifest, as well as the individual's strengths are all key to targeting treatment objectives and choosing treatment options.

Research has shown that early screening and pharmacological treatment of ADHD can reduce symptoms and improve general functioning by making adaptive strategies more effective; but it can also reduce the risk of a variety of problems, such as substance abuse, and the number of accidents, traumatic brain injuries and emergency room visits due to accidental injuries. As the therapeutic approach takes shape, it's important to have a frank discussion about the elements·that lead to choosing pharmacological treatment. This discussion should focus on issues like the primary effects desired and the risks involved in choosing not to treat ADHD.

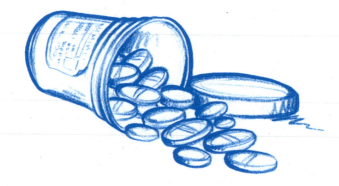

Set realistic objectives

Experts agree that treatment involving an ADHD medication is recommended if adaptive strategies are not effective enough, if the costs of the compensatory burden are disproportionate in terms of time and energy, or if there are major potential risks or impacts associated with ADHD symptoms.

ADHD medication activates certain areas of the brain, allowing an individual with ADHD to focus better. The primary effects of ADHD medication are associated with an improved ability to self-modulate. Effort and energy spent trying to "re-center" become more successful, making adaptive strategies more effective. Mental restlessness subsides, and affected persons have an easier time directing their thoughts despite the presence of distracting stimuli; this helps them be less scattered and stay concentrated. Forgetfulness is alleviated, and less time is wasted looking for missing objects. This "self-regulating" effect can also improve control of physical restlessness (hyperactivity) and help the individual take time before reacting, reducing associated impulsivity. Results start to better reflect the efforts made, and the chance of successfully completing projects increase. Self-esteem is gradually rebuilt. Individuals can access their personal resources, which allows them to flourish and reach their full potential.

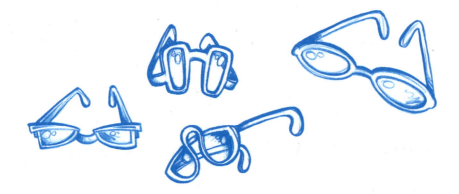

But, be careful! A pair of glasses helps you see better, but doesn't teach you to read; similarly, medication is not a cure-all. It isn't a motor that helps a person with ADHD start their day; it doesn't make tasks more interesting and doesn't magically help you organize a planner. A target for pharmological treatment should meet the **SMART** criteria: it should be **S**imple, **M**easurable, **A**ttainable in a **R**ealistic way within a set **T**ime frame. Here are a series of SMART objectives for treating ADHD: reduce the number of "careless mistakes;" improve sustained concentration, in spite of distracting stimuli; better control fidgeting; reduce restlessness; and improve the ability to wait one's turn and take time before acting. It's important to note that **academic results are neither a good indicator of an ADHD diagnosis nor a way to measure treatment efficacy**, because various other factors (apart from ADHD) can affect grades.

The different options for pharmalogical treatments for ADHD

The ideal pharmacological treatment would help significantly reduce the symptoms of ADHD and their impacts (primary effects) throughout the period targeted, and produce few undesireable impacts (secondary effects). It should also be easy to administer at a reasonable cost. Thanks to research advances, a number of different types of molecules and ways of releasing the active ingredient have appeared. However, the medications described in this chapter are not available everywhere, and it's important to note that a product can have different brand names and distinct indications, depending on the country.

Medication is part of a multimodal approach consisting of multiple strategies used in synergy. Medications approved for the treatment of ADHD result in **clinical improvement among 50% to 70% of persons affected**. Research has shown that psychostimulants can reduce ADHD symptoms in children over the age of six, adolescents and adults. Therapeutic effects of a lesser — but still very significant — degree have also been demonstrated for "non-stimulant" formulations. It should be noted that studies for some medications have focused mainly on young persons aged six to 17.

Regardless of the product chosen, any ADHD medication should be started at a low dose and adjusted on an individual basis. The clinician should consider the duration of the effect and adjust the interval between doses. Like glasses that correct vision only when they are worn, ADHD medication can only produce its effect when it is in your body. Some individuals may have a better response to one type of product than another, and there are no clinical or biological indicators that make it possible to determine the optimal treatment for each individual beforehand. To choose between therapeutic options, the doctor will also consider other problems that may be associated with ADHD such as anxiety, depression and substance abuse.

All the treatments that are currently known to be effective to reduce the intensity of ADHD symptoms improve noradrenaline and/or dopamine neurotransmission. These treatments function like putting a pair of "biological glasses" on the brain: they improve its ability to focus.

There are two classes of ADHD drugs: psychostimulants and non-psychostimulants. **Psychostimulants** act mainly by increasing the availability of dopamine in the synapse. Atomoxetine, viloxazine, guanfacine and clonidine all belong to the class of **non-psychostimulants**, but each has a distinct mechanism of action. Atomoxetine and viloxazine increase the availability of noradrenaline and, indirectly, dopamine in some regions of the brain, by blocking the noradrenaline reuptake pump. Guanfacine and clonidine mimic the effects of noradrenaline on the alpha-2a post-synaptic receptors. Clonidine has a more general effect, while guanfacine acts specifically on the alpha-2a subtype. Their different mechanisms of action may explain why these products can have different clinical effects.

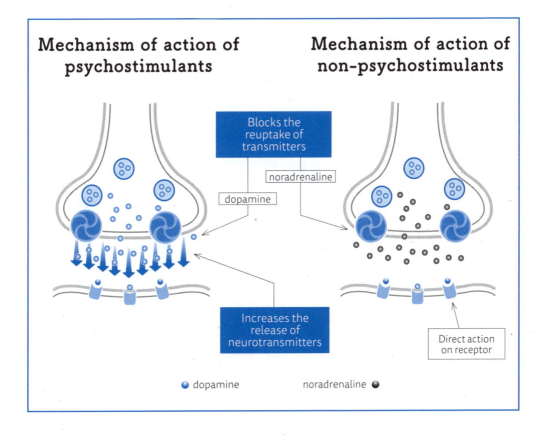

Mechanism of action of psychostimulants

Mechanism of action of non-psychostimulants

Blocks the reuptake of transmitters

noradrenaline

dopamine

Increases the release of neurotransmitters

Direct action on receptor

● dopamine   noradrenaline ●

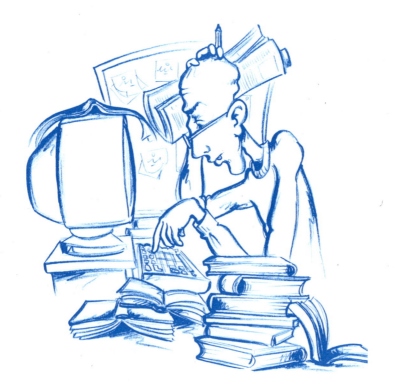

Psychostimulants

Psychostimulants include two families of drugs: **methylpheni-date**-based products and **amphetamine**-based products.

Some methylphenidate-based products contain just one form, dextro-methylphenidate (d-methylphenidate). Because dextro-methylphenidate is more effective than regular methylphenidate, the total daily doses (in milligrams) are lower. The duration of clinical effect of methylphenidate and its dextro form are similar.

The active ingredient in amphetamine-based psychostimulants is primarily dextro-amphetamine. These medications can be prescribed as a first therapeutic option and are not reserved for complex cases or for individuals whose symptoms endure despite trying other medications.

The onset of action of psychostimulants occurs rapidly, within hours of intake. The duration of the effect varies according to the drug's release mode. When the correct dosage is reached, clinical response is observed on a day that the medication has been taken. If the person does not take the medication, clinical effects cannot be observed. Psychostimulants are usually taken daily, but may also be used on an ad hoc basis, depending on therapeutic goals.

Release modes vary from drug to drug. Psychostimulants are available in **immediate release** (3- to 4-hour duration), **gradual release** (6- to 8-hour duration), and extended release (a duration of up to 12 hours or more, with a sustained effect over time that varies depending on the release mode).

Medication and modes of release

In order to better understand how a medication's mode of release can impact its clinical effects, here are three diagrams that illustrate the efficiency curve for different types of products. Note that the situations presented are a theoretical representation and do not correspond to a particular medication.

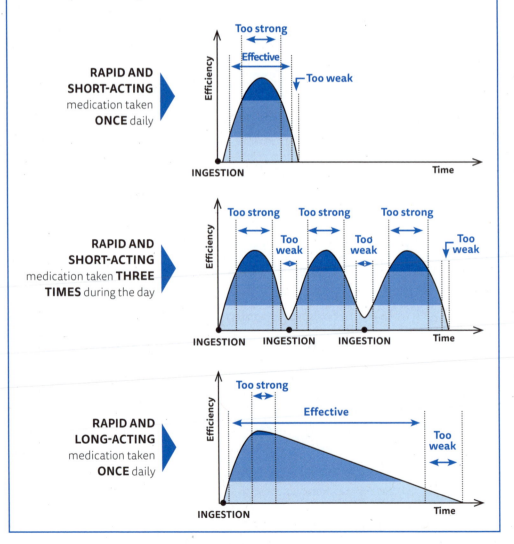

The amount of immediate versus delayed release, and the rate at which the psychostimulant reaches peak concentration before being eliminated from the body, can influence not only the duration of the drug's effect, but also the medication's clinical response (primary effects) and tolerability (side effects). For example, the duration of the desired effects may not match the individual's needs if the psychostimulant is released too slowly (late onset of efficacy) or if the amount available disappears too quickly (loss of efficacy before the period required). Similarly, adverse effects may be accentuated if the product is released at too rapid a rate.

Medical research is ongoing. Scientists are trying to develop innovative formulas to meet specific needs. In recent years, several new delivery mechanisms have been developed, including one that allows for a **delayed** release of the psychostimulant. Its effect begins approximately 8 hours after intake and continues for 12 hours. This type of drug may be useful for those who need a sustained therapeutic effect that begins early in the day. Since it must be taken the night before, timing is key to ensure good control of ADHD symptoms throughout the following day, from beginning to end.

Psychostimulants are available in a variety of delivery methods, including **capsules** (some whose contents can be sprinkled), tablets to be **swallowed**, **chewed** or that **dissolve rapidly**, and others in the form of a **liquid** containing **micro-granules in suspension**.

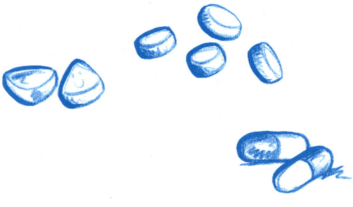

There is also a **transdermal patch** whose effects persist for several hours after removal, allowing the duration of effect to be adjusted according to when it is applied and removed.

When any given medication is being considered to help a person cope with ADHD and function to their full potential, the clinician and the person collaborate to define the areas of life being affected and to determine what periods of the day the medication would allow for better control of symptoms. The clinician also checks the person's ability to swallow tablets, which guides the form of psychostimulant chosen from among the many available.

Chewable tablets, fast-dissolving tablets, capsules that can be sprinkled or diluted in liquid, as well as patch and liquid formulations make it easier for people who have difficulty swallowing tablets.

Here are some examples of various release methods.

Multilayer-release methylphenidate

Multilayer-release methylphenidate allows for sustained clinical action over 10 to 12 hours or over 16 hours by initially releasing 40% or 20% of the active medication, followed by a more progressive release of the remaining 60% or 80%. This multilayer-granule release mechanism may be sensitive to pH levels in the digestive tract. Persons who have difficulty swallowing can sprinkle the contents of the capsule on their food.

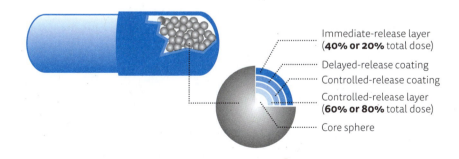

Immediate-release layer
(**40% or 20%** total dose)

Delayed-release coating
Controlled-release coating

Controlled-release layer
(**60% or 80%** total dose)

Core sphere

Methylphenidate tablet with an osmotic release oral system (OROS™)

The methylphenidate tablet with an osmotic release oral system (OROS™) pump technology immediately releases 22% of the total dose (in the coating), with the remainder released progressively in an upward curve using an integrated pump system that acts as a piston and expels the medicine from the tablet, providing a clinical effect that can last up to 12 hours. The duration of the effect may vary according to the speed of digestive transit. To ensure this mechanism of release, do not cut or chew the tablet.

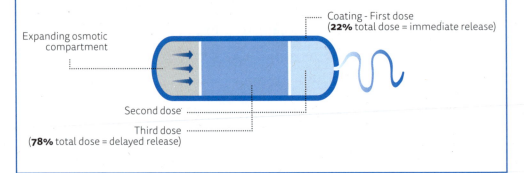

Coating - First dose
(**22%** total dose = immediate release)

Expanding osmotic compartment

Second dose

Third dose
(**78%** total dose = delayed release)

Lisdexamfetamine

Lisdexamfetamine (LDX) uses a different mode of release. In the medical jargon, it is known as a prodrug. The capsule is filled with a biologically inactive complex made up of dextroamphetamine coupled to an amino acid called lysine. Enzymes found in the digestive system and the blood break the link, allowing dextroamphetamine to be released progressively. This mechanism is not affected by digestive transit time or by pH, which may explain its day-to-day and person-to-person stability. The release profile is the same whether the product is ingested, snorted or injected. Studies have demonstrated clinical effects lasting 13 hours in children and adolescents and 14 hours in adults. Lisdexamfetamine is available both as a chewable tablet and a capsule whose contents are soluble in water, orange juice and yogurt.

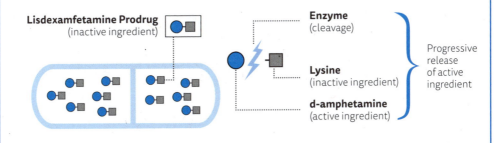

Mixed salts amphetamines

Mixed salts amphetamines contain four active ingredients, including dextroamphetamine. They are available in immediate-release tablets and two different types of extended-release capsules (double-bead and triple-bead formulations). The "long-acting" effect of this formulation is possible thanks to different types of coated granules. The triple-bead formulation permits an effect starting at 2 to 4 hours post-dose and lasting up to 16 hours and is planned for once-daily ADHD treatment for adults and children patients 13 and older. Here's an illustration of how the two-bead formulation works. Granules with less coating (50%) are digested more quickly and are activated first because of their immediate release.

Uncoated granule immediate release (**50%** total dose)

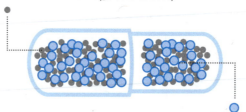

Coated granule delayed release (**50 %** total dose)

The body takes a certain amount of time to digest the other granules with thicker coating (50%), causing a second peak of release during the day, creating a prolonged effect of up to 12 hours. This release mechanism can be sensitive to stomach pH in the digestive tract. Individuals who have difficulty swallowing can sprinkle the contents of the capsule on their food.

Non-psychostimulants

Unlike with psychostimulants, nonstimulants need to be taken on a daily and sustained basis, since the clinical effect takes time to develop. This kind of ADHD medication therefore must be taken regularly to obtain and maintain a therapeutic effect. Patience is necessary as it can take one, two, or more weeks before it's possible to determine whether the dosage is right. Unlike psychostimulants, their therapeutic effect is relatively stable during the day, and they act somewhat like a base that allows for more continuous control of ADHD symptoms. This contrasts with the effects of psychostimulants, whose action has a distinct beginning and end and a specific duration, determined by the mode of release. The use of a nonstimulant can be particularly advantageous when ADHD symptoms need to be controlled from morning until late in the evening or nighttime, or for individuals for whom psychostimulants are unsuccessful due to severe secondary effects or insufficient clinical response despite optimized dosage.

Most people take **atomoxetine, viloxazine, guanfacine XR** or **clonidine XL** once a day, in a single morning or evening dose, but some tolerate it better when the dose is split and taken twice a day. Because guanfacine and clonidine can decrease heart rate and lower blood pressure, an abrupt interruption can cause a sharp rise in these parameters; therefore these medications should only be prescribed if the person can be sure to take them regularly, without acute interruptions or abrupt reductions in the dose.

"Off-label" medication

Some medications described in this chapter may be available in certain countries only because local health organizations have approved them for conditions other than ADHD. Other medications may be approved for the treatment of ADHD, but not for the age group of the individual in question. In some complex cases of ADHD, it may be possible to consider treatments that are approved for conditions other than ADHD if the conventional treatments have not worked and the functional impacts of ADHD are severe.

These cases involve "off-label" usage, and such an approach must be considered carefully, since the medication has not been approved for ADHD treatment in the region in question. An example: **modafinil** can help improve alertness among individuals with diurnal hypersomnolence, narcolepsy and shift-work sleep disorder. Clinical studies among adolescents and adults have demonstrated potential efficacy of modafinil for treatment of ADHD, but it is not approved specifically for the treatment of this disorder.

When an individual suffers from ADHD complicated by an associated anxiety or mood disorder, the doctor will prioritize the treatment of the most severe condition. It's also important to consider that ADHD medications may accentuate symptoms of anxiety and unbalance an underlying bipolar disorder. When ADHD is complicated by depression or anxiety, the doctor may suggest a therapeutic trial with **antidepressants** or **mood stabilizers** as monotherapy or in combination with a specific ADHD treatment. A small amount of research has been done to study the effects of these medications on persons with ADHD. Clinical studies with adolescents and adults have demonstrated a reduction in ADHD symptoms with **buproprion**, an antidepressant that can also be prescribed to help quit smoking. Among persons affected by mood disorders, mood stabilizers can alleviate extreme mood swings and may reduce impulsivity. However, these products have not been subject to clinical studies to assess their specific efficacy for emotional dysregulation associated with ADHD (hyperreactivity).

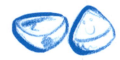

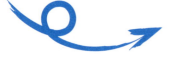

GOOD TO KNOW

What is a generic drug?

Some medications are also available in generic forms. To qualify as "generic," the drug must be declared "bioequivalent" based on standards set by the country where it is being marketed, following studies on a small group of healthy volunteers. These standards are based on a comparison between the release profiles of the generic medication and of the original product. Obviously, the generic drug should contain the same active substance as the original. The maximum concentration measured in the blood (Cmax) and the total quantity of product release (*area under the curve*, or AUC) must be similar to that of the original medication: i.e., within a given statistical range known as the "confidence interval."

In Canada, the required limits for these parameters are between 80% and 125% in comparison with the original product, and the time to reach the maximum concentration (Tmax) is not taken into account. Since the timing of the peak in blood concentration can vary between different generic drugs and the original product, the efficacy and tolerability may differ as well.

> Because bioequivalence doesn't always mean clini-
> cal equivalence, some people may report a difference
> in effect between the generic product and the origi-
> nal, while others may not.

Introducing and adjusting ADHD medication

The dosage for an ADHD medication is adjusted in the same way one adjusts the strength of a pair of glasses. It's important to proceed step by step to explore the effect of each dose. The universal rule in all cases is Start LOW and Go SLOW: the starting dose should be weak, then adjusted progressively, measuring clinical effects and detecting the occurrence of possible side effects. Working with the patient, their loved ones and other relevant persons, the doctor adapts the dosage, considering the therapeutic effects desired, the undesirable effects observed and the maximum recommended dose for each product. Experts agree that **the standard pharmacological treatment for ADHD is the same for children, adolescents and adults, but the maximum dose may vary according to age group**. For psychostimulants, there's no link between an individual's weight and the optimal therapeutic dose; for nonstimulants, a these two parameters may or may not be interrelated.

As with eyeglasses to correct myopia, the goal of pharmacological treatment of ADHD is to effectively control the symptoms when the person needs it – which often means throughout the day, every day. The method of administering the medication depends on its mode of release and duration of action. The timing of dosage is based on the drug's period of effectiveness and the portion of the day when the ADHD symptoms should be reduced.

Criteria to consider when choosing a medication

Clinical studies have shown that ADHD medications are effective and well-tolerated in most cases. According to the current literature, neither the profile of clinical symptoms (inattention vs. hyperactivity/ impulsivity) nor the genetic profile make it possible to predict the effect of pharmacological treatment of ADHD on a given individual.

The choice of treatment should be individualized to meet the specific needs of each person. The recommendations of Canadian experts at CADDRA, an organization for the evaluation and treatment of ADHD, are available on the site caddra.ca.

The doctor's role is to determine the right medication, its dose and the treatment protocol for each individual treated. In approaching these questions, the doctor should consider the following elements:

Efficacy

Psychostimulants are generally more effective than nonstimulants and are given priority as first-line therapy.

Duration of action

The "glasses for the brain" analogy is a good way to start a discussion with a person affected by ADHD and their loved ones, and to begin the search for the right duration of action.

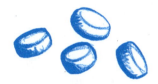

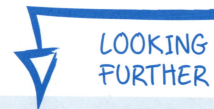

LOOKING FURTHER

Medication considerations

While less expensive, immediate-release (commonly called "short-acting") psychostimulants are associated with several problems:

- To maintain a clinical effect during the day, they should be taken every 3 or 4 hours. Tablets are also easy to misplace.

- Taking drugs outside of one's own home means losing an assurance of privacy. For example, some people may choose not to take their midday dose for fear that others may notice they need medication.

- The effect may be too powerful after taking a dose and may subside too quickly before the next dose. This can result in a roller-coaster sensation of effects, often labeled as peak-and-valley effects.

- Immediate-release psychostimulants are associated with a higher risk of misuse and abuse than extended-release products.

In light of all these factors, experts from CADDRA take the view that immediate-release psychostimulants should be used for second-line treatments or adjunctive therapies, and that extended-release psychostimulants should be used for first-line therapy.

Nonstimulants may successfully be used to control symptoms for 24 hours. They must be taken continuously and cannot be taken occasionally, on an as-needed base. According to CADDRA, these medications should be used for second-line treatment, in monotherapy or in combination with psychostimulants if there is a suboptimal response to the latter. In Canada, only guanfacine XL has been officially approved for ADHD treatment in co-administration with a psychostimulant when treatment with methylphenidate- and amphetamine-based psychostimulants has failed to adequately control ADHD in individuals under the age of 18.

Accessibility

The clinician should check whether the medication in question is available and indicated by the country's governmental authorities for the treatment of ADHD and for the individual's age group. It is also important to consider the cost of treatment (are the drugs covered by insurance?).

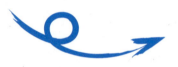 GOOD TO KNOW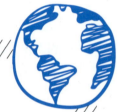

Medications around the world

The various products indicated for the treatment of ADHD globally are differentiated by their active ingredient and their mode of release. The type of release mechanism affects the method by which the product becomes available in the organism, the speed with which its action begins and ends and the duration of the effect. The commercial names, dosage and indications can vary from country to country.

In some countries, access to long-acting and once-daily medications is limited, either because the product isn't marketed in the region or because it isn't covered by insurance. However, experts recommend them as first-line treatment. Let's hope that effective treatment is soon available to all.

Ability to swallow a tablet

It is possible to teach someone techniques so they are better able to swallow a tablet. If the problem can't be overcome, consider the following alternatives:

- Chewable tablets
- Fast-dissolving tablets
- Capsules whose content can be sprinkled on food
- Prodrug that can be diluted in water, juice or yogurt
- Liquid formulations
- Transdermal patches

N.B.: Administering the drug in liquid form can also be a good option when a very precisely adjusted dosing is required.

When the presence of another condition complicates ADHD treatment

It can be difficult to treat ADHD when other mental or health problems, particularly cardiovascular risks, are present. CADDRA's experts provide guidance to doctors in a complete chapter on the subject in the Canadian ADHD guidelines (visit caddra.ca).

One recommendation is a step-by-step approach for ADHD with other psychiatric problems. To summarize, ADHD treatment in individuals who have already suffered from psychotic disorders or bipolar effective disorder needs the supervision of a medical specialist, as taking ADHD medication can unbalance these underlying conditions.

One recommendation is a step-by-step approach when concommittant psychiatric problems are present with ADHD. As taking ADHD medication can unbalance psychotic disorders or bipolar affective disorder, the treatment for individuals with ADHD who also suffer from those conditions requires the supervision of a medical specialist.

When ADHD is associated with an anxiety or depressive disorder, the doctor will prioritize treating the most severe or impairing problem first, following the principles that guide the therapy of this specific disorder, while assessing closely the evolution of the other conditions.

ADHD treatment for persons with drug addiction is complex and often requires a mixed approach that involves reducing the drug or alcohol problem while treating the underlying ADHD. This is especially relevant in cases where ADHD symptoms interfere with the Substance Use Disorder.

GOOD TO KNOW

Beware of the risks of misuse!

Using medication to reduce specific ADHD symptoms can have an indirect impact: it can cut down on the excessive time and energy spent on compensatory strategies. This can ease secondary fatigue caused by ADHD.

This is not the same target as trying to gain more energy overall in order to merely mask the symptoms of fatigue. In this respect, the risk of misuse and the potential for abuse must be part of the conversation on psychostimulants. People taking a psychostimulant may be asked by friends to share their medication so they can "study better" or "stay awake longer." This phenomenon is called "diversion," and it's an example of misuse of this type of medication. Anyone who uses a stimulant to mask their fatigue or improve their ability to pay attention in order to compensate for adverse effects of overwork or an unhealthy lifestyle is taking this kind of treatment for the wrong reasons. It is unwise to take any medication that has not been prescribed to you specifically. Anyone who thinks they require ADHD treatment should discuss this with their doctor.

Certain street drugs are taken abusively for their stimulating and euphoric effects. These effects are produced when the receptors in the "pleasure center" of the brain are bombarded with dopamine. This is the case for stimulants like cocaine, methamphetamine and speed. Don't confuse these drugs with the psychostimulants prescribed for ADHD; these medications do not produce this kind of effect when taken as prescribed. However, a significant energizing or euphoric effect may occur with these medications if they are ingested in excessive quantities (overdose) or if they are snorted or injected in order to bypass the digestion stage. If a person affected by ADHD or

→

those around them are likely to misuse or abuse the medication, it is recommended to favor a prescription of a nonstimulant or of a psychostimulant for which the extended-release formulation makes it harder to transform into a substance that can be snorted or injected.

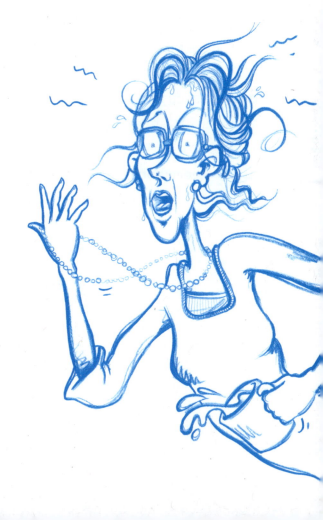

Managing side effects of medication

Every medication can produce unwanted side effects. The goal during treatment is to determine the optimal therapeutic dose to create a balance in which the desired primary effects outweigh the unwanted side effects. Some strategies can help reduce side effects. For instance, the effects of a medication with an extended-release mechanism are sometimes better tolerated than those with a fast release or a short action. The appearance of ADHD medication side effects may also be reduced by starting off with a weak dose taken regularly, then increasing the dose progressively following the "Start LOW, Go SLOW" principle. The body tends to become accustomed to side effects, while the therapeutic effects remain constant.

ADHD medications are generally well-tolerated. For some, however, the "effective and tolerated" zone may be narrower. In such cases, striking a balance between "not enough" and "too much" stimulation can be a tricky endeavor.

Difficult balance
Catecholamine levels (dopamine and noradrenaline)

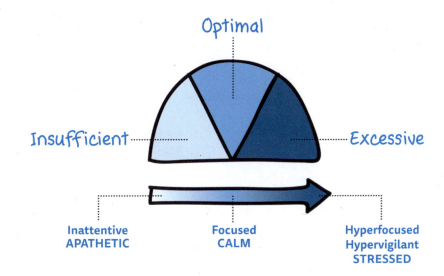

Persons whose ADHD is accompanied by other problems (an Anxiety Disorder, Mood Disorder — e.g., Bipolar Disorder — Autism Spectrum Disorder, intellectual impairment or an underlying neurological condition) often report greater sensitivity to hyperstimulation-like side effects such as hypervigilance, anxiety or restlessness.

When a person presents uncomfortable side effects, it is important to speak with a health care professional and explore whether other elements may be contributing to the unwanted side effects. Caffeine and nicotine also act as stimulants, and can therefore exacerbate side effects of ADHD medication.

TIPS FOR REDUCING THE INTENSITY OF SIDE EFFECTS

Some who take a medication to treat ADHD may notice a better result with one type of medication over another. It is important to thoroughly discuss the positive and negative effects of any medication with your doctor. The doctor may consider changing the active ingredient or the release mechanism if unwanted side effects persist or if the therapeutic effect is unsatisfactory. It is essential not to try to adjust your medication yourself, without discussing it with a health professional. If you have questions about treatments that are available, ask your doctor, nurse or pharmacist for more information.

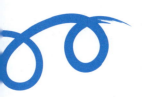

DIFFICULTY SLEEPING

People with ADHD often have difficulty sleeping, even without taking ADHD medication. They may find it hard to go to bed because they need to move or their agitated thoughts prevent them from settling down. Some seek stimulation from video games, television or the Internet, and lose track of passing time. Others procrastinate to avoid going to bed, even if they feel the warning signs of sleep. Many report that they find it hard to get up in the morning and feel jet-lagged. While some people find that their medication relieves their evening restlessness, others find it makes them too alert to fall asleep.

General advice

Here are some sleep hygiene tips that can help improve sleep. They are not specifically formulated for persons affected by ADHD or taking medication, and are frequently recommended to insomniacs by sleep specialists.

➡ Create a calm and comfortable environment to facilitate sleep.

➡ Use your bed only for sleep. If you have insomnia, don't read, watch television or do homework or office tasks in bed.

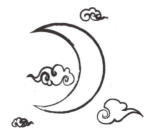

- ➡ Try to set healthy goals and aim for a reasonable bedtime and a reasonable time to get up in the morning.

- ➡ Develop a routine that gradually leads to sleep.

- ➡ Avoid overstimulation, coffee and other stimulants in the evening.

- ➡ Reduce brightness at night be turning off all screens at least 60 minutes before your planned bedtime.

- ➡ If sleep doesn't come after 20 or 30 minutes, get up and do a neutral activity that leads to mental fatigue, such as reading, until you're able to fall asleep.

- ➡ Avoid spending time in bed in the morning and taking naps during the day, which can disrupt the sleep cycle.

- ➡ Do physical activity during the day, but avoid it in the two hours before bedtime if it has too much of a stimulating effect.

Sometimes, nonrestorative sleep may be an indication of anxiety, depression or other problems, such as sleep apnea.

Sleep and medication

When medication seems to be responsible for disturbed sleep, here are two solutions to consider:

- ➡ Take the medication earlier.

- ➡ Talk to your doctor about the possibility of changing the type of medication or mode of release.

LOSS OF APPETITE OR NAUSEA

Some people may find that the medication prescribed to reduce ADHD symptoms also reduces appetite. Most of the time, this side effect is mild and temporary, but it may be more severe and persistent. If a loss of appetite is being experienced, but the treatment is very helpful, the person may decide with their doctor to maintain the medication. Here are some tips that may be useful for this type of situation. In more complex cases of appetite loss, it is recommended to consult a nutritionist.

➡ Take the medication with or after a meal.

➡ Eat at a fixed time, take smaller portions and eat more when your appetite returns.

➡ In addition to daily meals, eat nutritious snacks at regular intervals, even in the evenings. Vary the flavors and foods; opt for cheeses, yogurt (as rich as possible), whole grain cereals, smoothies with fruit and yogurt, milkshakes, muffins (be sure that their protein content is higher than their sugar content).

➡ Avoid "taking the edge off" your appetite by nibbling or having drinks between meals and regular snacks. Watch out especially for juice, energy drinks and soft drinks, which are literally appetite suppressants and give your brain the illusion that you're full.

When reducing portions or if you're losing weight, be sure to compensate (increase energy intake with "good calories") using the following strategies:

➡ Add milk powder (skim milk or certain infant formulas for young children), 35% cream or different cheeses into soups and sauces.

➡ Add baby cereals into different recipes and dishes: homemade muffins, pancake batter, oatmeal and certain sauces.

➡ Add non-hydrogenated margarine or canola oil into vegetable dishes, sauces and pastas.

➡ Add gratin dishes or garnish fruits or desserts with 35% whipped cream.

Some may choose to add dietary supplements to certain recipes. Certain insurance companies and mutuals will reimburse specific dietary supplements if they are prescribed by a doctor under the right circumstances. Talk to your doctor to find out more.

DRY MOUTH

➡ Chew sugarless gum.

➡ Eat sugarless candies.

➡ Drink water.

➡ Have good dental hygiene. This is especially important if you have dry mouth, because saliva helps protect against cavities.

HEADACHES OR MUSCLE TENSION

Headaches are often temporary, mild, and associated with a change in dosage.

➡ Take acetaminophen-containing medications if necessary.

Muscle tension can lead to tightness of the jaw and difficulty breathing deeply. This phenomenon may indicate that the dose is too high, which means that the treatment should be reviewed with a health care professional.

INCREASE OR DECREASE IN HEART RATE AND BLOOD PRESSURE

Psychostimulants, atomoxetine, and viloxazine can increase heart rate and blood pressure (BP), while guanfacine and clonidine can lower them. It's important to be cautious and check for a personal or family history of heart problems.

➡ Measure pulse and BP, particularly when changing dosage. For more rigorous control, use a tensiometer at a pharmacy, or buy one for the home.

➡ If BP is too high, avoid coffee and other stimulants. If BP is too low, increase the intake of liquids and salt. Consult a doctor if these parameters stay beyond the normal range for the person's age.

MOOD CHANGES

Feelings of feverishness, irritability or anxiety

It's important to distinguish the symptoms of an underlying anxiety disorder from the appearance of the side effects of overstimulation, a potential side effect associated with ADHD medication.

➡ Avoid coffee, tea and other stimulants such as chocolate or energy drinks.

➡ Talk to a doctor about the possibility of changing the type of medication or its mode of release, and consider using a non-psychostimulant.

➡ Consider a specific treatment for the underlying anxiety disorder, if symptoms of anxiety exist before ADHD medication is introduced.

Dullness, hyperfocus

A treatment with the proper dose should allow a person's creativity to be expressed and help him or her to see projects through to completion. An excessive dosage, on the other hand, could lead to feeling a loss of spontaneity or emotionally blunted, as if the task at hand is all that matters ("zombie effect"). The appearance of depression, sometimes accompanied by dark thoughts or ideation, has been described in rare cases. Reactions like these are signs that the medication isn't adjusted properly, and a health professional should be consulted to decrease the dosage or change the type of treatment.

CHANGE IN ENERGY LEVEL

Sensation of fatigue or lethargy

This type of sensation may be transient. If it persists, it may be a sign that the dosage is too high.

➡ Talk to your doctor about reducing the dosage or changing the type of medication.

Energy peak at the start of a dose, followed by a "crash" or intense feeling of fatigue at the end of the dose (under psychostimulant medication)

This type of sensation may indicate that the dosage is too high or that the effect of the psychostimulant is wearing off too quickly.

➡ **Do not use psychostimulants to mask fatigue or boost energy!**

➡ Discuss with your doctor the possibility of changing the type of medication or delivery method, or consider using a non-psychostimulant medication.

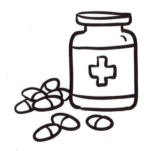

The importance of continued monitoring

ADHD treatment integrates an individualized, multimodal, multi-disciplinary and progressive approach, and taking medication requires medical monitoring. This should be more intensive during periods of dosage adjustment, but visits can be farther apart later on. Plan for periods of reevaluation during times of transition, and regular follow-ups for medication.

Many people discontinue their treatment due to oversight, failure to renew a prescription or giving up on medical follow-ups. These unexpected discontinuations don't follow a therapeutic goal.

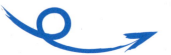 GOOD TO KNOW /////////////

USEFUL LITTLE TIPS
Make a note of appointment dates!
Persons affected by ADHD are prone to procrastination and may tend to keep postponing doctor's appointments, or miss appointments because they forget them or show up late. To make sure you get regular medical monitoring, it is strongly recommended that you make your next appointment as

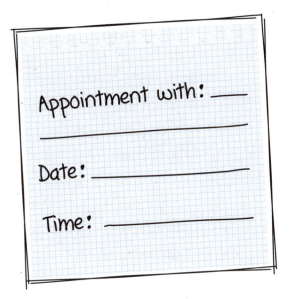

you're leaving the doctor's office. Make a note of the time and date in your planner and, if necessary, ask someone you trust to remind you the day before.

Remember to take your medication!

- Use a pill dispenser or Dispill™ blister pack system.
- Make a note or set an alarm as a reminder.
- Keep "emergency" pills in strategic places such as your purse or glove compartment; Store the medication in a secure place that is inaccessible to children.

Medication: an evolving strategy

Deciding to take medication doesn't mean signing a lifetime contract! When considering decreasing or discontinuing treatment, it is important to plan the right moment, to continue medical monitoring with your doctor and to reassess a possible resumption of pharmacological treatment based on the evolution of symptoms.

Here are some situations in which a planned reduction or discontinuation of ADHD medication may be worth considering:

Disabling side effects

In the presence of persistant side effects, the doctor may suggest reducing the dosage or discontinuing treatment during targeted periods – for example, weekends and holidays – or trying another medication with a different active ingredient or mode of release.

Insufficient efficacy

When treatments do not result in significant clinical improvement in spite of optimized dosage, it is perfectly appropriate to reduce the treament, and ultimately to discontinue it (on a doctor's recommendation and with continued monitoring). Before deciding that an effect is insufficient, don't forget to analyze the elements that may aggravate manifestations of ADHD, such as a lack of sleep or an excessively busy schedule. Sometimes reducing dosage or discontinuing treatment helps a person realize that the treatment was actually effective and leads them to start it again.

Pregnancy and breastfeeding

We don't know very much about the effects of ADHD medication on the fetus or breastfed infants. Therefore, it is strongly recommended for women of childbearing age to use effective contraception when taking these medications. If a pregnancy is planned, it is important to speak to your doctor. The decision whether or not to discontinue ADHD treatment must be made on an individual basis, by evaluating the risks for the mother as well as the potential risks for the future child.

Clinical improvement

In cases where the person seems to present no current manifestations of ADHD, it is recommended to regularly reevaluate the need to maintain the medication and to start by considering reducing the dosage, leading up to an eventual discontinuation.

Whatever the treatment options chosen, it is a good idea to periodically assess their relevance by looking at their efficacy (primary effects), the side effects of the medication and the cost of the compensatory burden linked to the extra time and energy needed to implement the necessary adaptive strategies.

The objective does not change: to allow each person to find which "pair of glasses" fits them better so they can reach their full potential!

Two years ago I learned that my problems were associated with what is called ADHD. All my life, I instinctively found and applied tricks to reduce the impact of ADHD in my daily life. Understanding ADHD has helped me to develop new strategies. It takes enormous effort and the results aren't always as big as the energy invested. I forget to look at my planner. I lose my fifth set of keys. I'm often late for work and scattered in handling my tasks. Medication helps my brain work better. The fog lifts and my ideas — and my efforts — become organized. I'm less stressed because I'm more functional. My self-esteem is better: I can dare to create and take on projects and I finish what I start. My friends say that they feel like I'm more "there". For me, medication has made a difference. It makes me sad when people who are not well informed oppose medication. If they only knew!

Manon, age 45

CHECKLIST FOR STEP 5

Let's review the main points presented in this section:

❯ There's no such thing as a miracle medication. Treatment should be carried out under medical supervision.

❯ The pharmacological treatment approach starts with clarifying the diagnosis, and identifying targets and therapeutic approaches to address the impact and the compensatory burden.

❯ The medications available to treat ADHD are psychostimulants and non-psychostimulants.

❯ Psychostimulants act mainly by increasing the availability of dopamine in the synapse by blocking its reuptake and by increasing its release. Methylphenidate-based and amphetamine-based psychostimulants are available as immediate- or delayed-release products.

❯ Atomoxetine and viloxazine are non-psychostimulants that enable increased availability of noradrenaline in the synapse by blocking its reuptake.

> Guanfacine, a non-psychostimulant, imitates the action of noradrenaline acting selectively on the alpha-2a receptors, while clonidine, another non-stimulant, has a similar but less specific action.

> It is important to target treatment objectives and to reassess the effects during follow-up. The overall target is to allow the person to live better with ADHD and develop to his or her full potential.

> Medications act like "biological glasses for the brain," helping to reduce ADHD symptoms and allowing coping mechanisms to work more effectively.

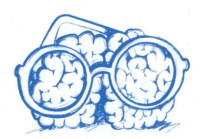

Considerations for the future

I have the privilege of being surrounded by extraordinary people who are dealing with ADHD, both in my professional and my personal life. Colleagues, friends, family, athletes, students, artists, entrepreneurs, professionals, tradespersons, parents – no matter how our paths cross, I learn from them, and grow from having met them. Being able to guide these people, to give them tools to live better with ADHD and to help them flourish is a source of inspiration that motivates me to give back. A life journey with ADHD has many challenging moments. The important thing is to try, to accept slips and falls sometimes, and to always try again. Every journey is unique, colored by each person's distinctive personality and the personality of those around them. The keys to success are: **understand**, **adapt and change**, **be resilient**, **persevere**, **move** and **act**, **tame** your emotions and your ADHD, **find your passion**, **have fun**, **surround yourself** with the right people, **treat** yourself and your loved ones **with care and kindness**, **believe in yourself**, **be daring** and **be proud** of your difference as you **explore** strategies and find the right "pair of glasses" for you.

Our understanding of ADHD is advancing steadily. Research is in full swing, services are becoming available, and we know more about ADHD from childhood to adulthood. Myths are being challenged. People living with the condition, and their loved ones, are increasingly better equipped to cope with ADHD, and more and more treatments options are available to them.

By understanding ADHD better, you can, if you choose, act as a catalyst in your community and contribute to the development of a better help network for people living with ADHD in your own way. For these people and their loved ones, I deeply hope that this book serves as a stepping stone to the personal fulfillment that we all desire.

Annick Vincent
Psychiatrist

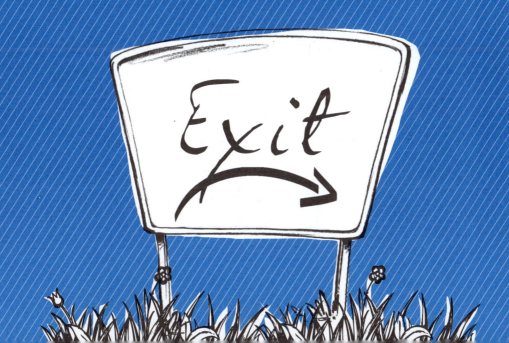

Resources and references

My Brain Needs Glasses: ADHD explained to kids

Tom is 8 years old and coping with Attention Deficit Hyperactivity Disorder (ADHD). Through his journal, he opens the door to his daily life, allowing kids, parents and others to better understand and deal with ADHD. Funny and imaginative, the story told by this endearing character will take readers into a world that has its own share of challenges that are anything but imaginary. Filled with useful tips and practical advice for living better with ADHD, this book is an indispensable tool that will answer myriad questions for young and old alike.

VINCENT, A. *My Brain Needs Glasses: ADHD explained to kids*, Juniper Publishing, 2022.

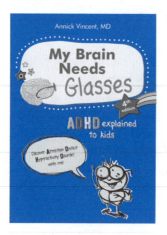

Also available in French and Korean

VINCENT, A. *Mon cerveau a ENCORE besoin de lunettes: le TDAH chez les adolescents et les adultes*, Montreal, Les Éditions de l'Homme, 2022.

VINCENT, A. *Mon cerveau a besoin de lunettes: le TDAH expliqué aux enfants*, Montreal, Les Éditions de l'Homme, 2022.

Tools, practical tips,
videos and lists of ADHD resources

Visit the ADHD website developed by the author, Dr. Annick Vincent, to learn more tips and tricks and to find out about available resources: attentiondeficit-info.com

Imprimé chez Marquis Imprimeur inc. sur du Rolland Enviro.
Ce papier contient 100% de fibres postconsommation,
est fabriqué avec un procédé sans chlore
et à partir d'énergie biogaz.